Stop Battling Disease
and
Start Building Wellness

Your Guide to Extraordinary Health

Stop Battling Disease
and
Start Building Wellness

Your Guide to Extraordinary Health

Tonijean Kulpinski, CBHC, BCHP, AADP,
Board-Certified Holistic Drugless Practitioner

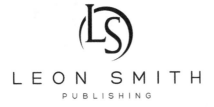

LEON SMITH
PUBLISHING

LeonSmithPublishing.com

Dedication

I dedicate this book:

First and foremost, I thank you, Lord, for giving me an entirely new life and the knowledge and wisdom to share my story and journey.

To my family, for putting up with me when I yelled and chased them out of the room while I was writing.

To my dear husband, for being right by my side each and every step of the way.

To my precious daughter, Michaela, for being so patient with her needs while I wrote. Michaela, Mommy loves you more than you can ever imagine. My baby girl, you are the air that I breathe.

Acknowledgments

I thank my amazing mother for giving me the encouragement that I needed to believe in myself.

I thank my dear sister, Fran, who always finds the time to support me no matter what.

My incredible brother, Richard, thank you for encouraging and believing in me although you're so many miles away.

My wonderful niece, Michelle, the most selfless person I know: I thank you for always building me up exactly where I need to be.

My dog, Peanut, I thank you for your submission when you wanted to play, and I needed to finish a chapter.

I thank my dear friends: Nicole Roberts for showing me how to put my knowledge into a book, and Christine Felicello for giving me the support that I needed to move forward.

My dear friend, Angela Wallace, I could not have accomplished this without you.

Lennis Giansante, thank you for holding my head up high when I was sick and scared; you knew exactly what God had in store for my future.

Kathy Meroney, you are a true-life angel, and I thank you for blessing me with your loyal and loving friendship.

I thank everyone else for supporting me through their interest in my nutritional knowledge.

Last, I want to acknowledge Keith and Maura Leon. You have been the most amazing people through this journey. You not only accepted me initially, but have worked hard answering all my questions and concerns. Together with your team, you made me feel such assurance and peace. I couldn't be happier with the final layout. I thank each of you for working diligently over the last year, making this dream a reality. I can honestly say that I love each of you for the gifts that you have, and for touching my life in many ways. I've learned so much through this journey. What an honor it truly is to be a part of your team. Thank you with every bit of my heart for giving me the opportunity to touch the lives of those who need it and for taking in an amateur writer who hoped to become a best seller.

Contents

Introduction

If a flower does not bloom, we fix the environment in which it grows, not the flower.
— Alexander Den Heijer

We must stop battling disease and start building wellness.

I wrote this book for many reasons — first and foremost is the loss of so many lives each day from cancer and other devastating diseases. Unfortunately, as most of us have witnessed firsthand, loved ones suffer from various conventional treatments and therapies that make many promises. I have heard too many times the words: *she has lost her battle,* or *he put up a good fight.*

Are we living longer, or are we dying longer?

We are currently in a major health crisis. Illnesses of all kinds have created an epidemic of sick people. Statistics show that 70 percent of the human race is overweight, and the other 30 percent is morbidly obese. Childhood obesity has become a serious health concern.

We are overfed, undernourished, and we are starving for real, whole-food nutrition. About 20 percent of what we eat keeps us alive, and the other 80 percent keeps the doctor alive.

We humans have brought about the severe destruction of our beautiful planet. God has given us every seed-bearing plant for our food on the face of this whole Earth (Genesis 1:29 NET), yet with human ingenuity, we have genetically modified the structure of our food, resulting in severe sickness and massive ecological damage.

Ten years ago, the incidence of cancers in the United States was one out of every five individuals. Five years ago, it was one in three. Now, *one in every two people* are diagnosed with cancer. Fourteen thousand U.S. children are diagnosed with rare types of cancers annually and more than half of those children die.

In the last sixty-plus years, the world of Western medicine is still removing body parts, radiating, and using chemotherapy; yet statistics prove that most people diagnosed with cancer will die within five years.

The medical establishment still claims they are closer to a cure. But the cure has been around longer than the cause, and it's not found in conventional therapies that cause more individual self-destruction. The cure can be found in organic, whole, unprocessed, God-created food.

We must first treat the patient, not the disease. The body has innate wisdom of self-healing, but to achieve that, we must first stop *battling* disease and start *building* wellness.

The Almighty Physician has stated clearly in scripture guidelines and principles how to care for our physical bodies. If we follow these guidelines and principles, we will have less incidence of disease.

As followers of God's word, I believe we are held accountable to take care of our physical bodies as living sacrifices. Our bodies are the temples of our living God. We must care for them as well as caring for the land. This is our reasonable act of worship.

Together we are one. We have witnessed this world become toxic—the soil depleted, the oceans poisoned, animals abused for food, plants drenched with chemicals, birds and bees traveling in mass confusion from toxic overload. As a result, we have an epidemic of sick people.

I wholeheartedly believe that together we have the power to change this rapid mass destruction. We must first recognize that greed has taken the place of true peace and harmony.

> *Behold, I will bring it health and cure, and I will cure them, and will reveal unto them the abundance of peace and truth.*
> —Jeremiah 33:6 KJV

The earth produces the most amazing and well-needed medicine that is designed so perfectly to satisfy all our nutritional requirements. We need to stop dispensing our health out of a drug container, because the cures have been around longer than the cause. Nature within itself feeds us, not humans and technology.

I believe that true love has been removed from the equation of perfect health and replaced with greed. I also believe that we must open our eyes and take a good look at the magnificence of God's creations all around us. We are intricately connected, and we all receive life and instruction from the same source. This is the critical message that has been stolen from us, yet it's been right here all along, hidden in plain sight.

> *In the midst of the street of it, and on either side of the river, was there the tree of life, which bare twelve manner of fruits, and yielded her fruit every month: and the leaves of the tree were for the healing of the nations.*
> —Revelation 22:2 KJV

I have absorbed much information within the last decade pertaining to health and healing, which has contributed to an incredible base of knowledge. More important, however, is my inner wisdom that tells me in my heart who I truly am. I used both the knowledge and wisdom, along with my personal journey, to put together this book in the hope of changing many lives. It is my passion to continue to be the best version of myself so that you can be the best version of yourself.

I believe my dream is my mission and gift from God. It is my passion and purpose as I have dedicated my life to help restore the health of God's people — one life at a time.

Whether you are suffering from a debilitating medical condition, dealing with uncomfortable symptoms, or looking for prevention, may this book bring to you the answers that will unlock your God-given ability to live the life of better health the way you were meant to live. Your body is naturally equipped with everything it needs to live well.

As you embark on your healing journey, I hope you are encouraged by my personal story as well as the wealth of nutritional information that I have put together for each of you on your path to great health.

In Jesus' name, I pray the blessings of amazing health are bestowed upon each of you and your loved ones from the top of your head to the soles of your feet.

> *Dear friend, I pray that in every way you may prosper and enjoy good health, as your soul also prospers.*
> —3 John 1: 2 BSB

CHAPTER ONE

My Personal Testimony

Indeed, we felt we had received the sentence of death. But this happened that we might not rely on ourselves but on God who raises the dead.
— 2nd Corinthians 1:9 NIV

I am humble, as I learned the message of health the hard way. I was one of those teenage girls who struggled with her weight. My weight would go up and down, sometimes too far down. I would starve myself to fit into the latest fashion, only to regain it from nutritional starvation. I would yo-yo diet as a way of life, climbing up and down the scale, which would cause me to lose bone and muscle mass. As I approached my twenties and thirties, this pattern of life continued and my health suffered.

At the age of eighteen, I became a hairstylist and continued these unhealthy dietary patterns. By the time I was twenty-eight, I owned a beauty salon and worked as a heavy-duty colorist, breathing in many toxic chemicals and not eating properly. I had panic attacks, severe digestive issues, and drastic weight fluctuations. At one point I wasn't able to hold down much food.

I also had thyroid problems, chronic migraines, gallbladder issues, dizzy spells, bone loss, severe blood sugar issues, and a diagnosis of kidney cancer.

The diagnosis of kidney cancer was definitely the scariest wakeup call for me. Medical treatment was all I knew at the time, so on March 11, 2008, I had my left kidney removed. Thank goodness the cancer was *nonmetastatic,* or isolated, meaning there were no cancer cells anywhere else in the body. The pathology report indicated that there were traces of hair dye in my kidney that caused the cancer, a direct result of my profession.

I was so scared; I did not know where to turn and prayed that God would give me back my life. I continued to suffer from many of the symptoms that were mentioned above. Two days after the surgery, I began praying for God to give me a sign that would lead me into what I believed would heal me.

Although at that time I did not have much nutritional knowledge, I knew that just by removing an organ that hosted cancer, we were not removing the *cause.*

In the beginning of my search for an answer, my husband and I had gone to a local health food store where I had bumped into a bookshelf and knocked a book on the floor. As I bent down to pick up the book, I felt intense heat radiating off that book and into my hands. I knew as soon as I touched the book that it was the sign from God that would lead me to my new life. The book, *The Maker's Diet* by Jordan S. Rubin, changed my life forever as I began my healing journey.

Through Jordan's book, the Lord showed me guidelines and principles to heal my body that are stated clearly in scripture. I never knew that the Bible was a manual for health; I had thought it was only for spiritual needs. I started incorporating the biblically based food and lifestyle program into my life 100 percent.

My body immediately began to heal from all the various health issues that plagued me. In the beginning of the biblically based program, I had gone through a detox. My body started purging what I believed was years of toxicity. My headaches, digestive problems, and blood glucose issues disappeared. Over a short period of time I was totally disease-free and living a level of extraordinary health that I had never known existed.

The Lord then told me, "I have restored your health and I want you to dedicate your life as the vessel to guide my children to restore their health."

I was empowered by this command from my Lord and Savior. I then wanted to share this message with others and help transform this nation and world in the way God had healed me.

I began by studying with the Biblical Health Institute, founded by Jordan Rubin, and was certified as a Biblical Health Coach. I learned biblical principles that are stated clearly in scripture that pertained to health and healing. I incorporated these life-giving services into my new wellness practice that was once a chemical-laden hair salon. I placed people on life-giving paths to health and wellness according to God's way.

I studied as many holistic health programs as I could that relied on biblical nutrition. I then studied at the world's largest nutrition school, The Institute for Integrative Nutrition. There I learned well over one hundred dietary theories; the connection between nature, the human body, and mind; and how to take my practice to a level beyond what I could ever imagine.

I have not only been blessed with total restoration in my body, but I also am blessed to be able to share this information with many others and to see their transformations. I was once trapped inside a jail cell — my body — now I live in extraordinary health all the time.

I could not wait another minute to begin delivering to millions of people the message of health that restored me. They were suffering needlessly. I began teaching holistic nutrition at a local college for adult enrichment. I have appeared on Trinity Broadcast Network's (TBN) *Joy in our Town* and *Doctor-to-Doctor*, discussing health and wellness.

God has used me as a transmitter of health and wellness in which I unlock people's God-given ability to heal themselves. I educate my clients about how to stop battling disease and start building wellness.

When I asked the Lord to give me back my life, He never did; He gave me an entirely new one.

Today I am 100 percent disease- and prescription-drug-free, and each day I reap the blessings of extraordinary health the way we were truly designed to be. I am the proud owner of Heaven On Earth Healing Center, Inc., where I place anyone whom God sends me, with any form of sickness, on the pathway to total health and healing.

I would never change my past, because it was the journey to my present and future.

> *You intended to harm me, but God intended it for good to accomplish what is now being done, the saving of many lives.*
>
> — Exodus 50:20 NIV

I love the path that God has placed me on. I have the opportunity each day to see the hidden health messages behind every life that enters my practice and, therefore, deliver the real truth of health and healing that is saving the lives of many. Removing people from the ravages of sickness and the bondage of the sick-care industry is so very rewarding.

It is my mission to educate God's people about the amazing benefits of real, whole, organic food. I believe that this is the medicine that prevents disease and restores health. The answer to great health is not the damaging immune-altering effects of prescription drugs and vaccines. The answer is the reconnection of nature and the human body. I live my passion simply because it is my purpose.

Sickness is not a death sentence, but a life sentence: an opportunity to transform your own health to be a testament to inspire others.

CHAPTER TWO

Principles of Biblical Nutrition

Great health is not about deprivation and restriction; great health is about abundance.

I believe that the Bible is a manual for health and happiness. The Bible was given to us by the Creator, our loving God, to save His people from the ravages of disease. This manual has guidelines and principles that teach us how to take care of our bodies — which are temples — so we can live the life of extraordinary health we were created to live.

> *Therefore, I urge you, brothers and sisters, in view of God's mercy, to offer your bodies as a living sacrifice, holy and pleasing to God – this is your true and proper worship.*
> — Romans 12:1 NIV

> *If you listen carefully to the LORD your God and do what is right in his eyes, if you pay attention to his commands and keep all his decrees, I will not bring on you any of the diseases I brought on the Egyptians, for I am the LORD, who heals you.*
> — Exodus 15:26 NIV

Eating More Fruits and Veggies Is Exactly What the Almighty Physician Ordered

Do you not know that your bodies are temples of the Holy Spirit, who is in you, whom you have received from God? You are not your own; you were bought at a price. Therefore, honor God with your body.

—1 Corinthians 6:19–20 NIV

Our bodies are temples, and their nourishment will affect the way we think and perform. The foods we eat transform our minds, and our minds transform our bodies. Humans have forgotten that real food is medicine, and that God has provided for us on all levels.

"Please test your servants for ten days: Give us nothing but vegetables to eat and water to drink. Then compare our appearance with that of the young men who eat the royal food, and treat your servants in accordance with what you see."

So, he agreed to this and tested them for ten days. At the end of the ten days, they looked healthier and better nourished than any of the young men who ate the royal food.

—Daniel 1:12–15 NIV

The benefits of fruits and vegetables are endless, and therefore in this chapter you will learn about God's bountiful creations of every seed-bearing plant. However, I do encourage you to consume food only in the form God has intended. Organic is the origin of our food and therefore spares us from the toxic overload and burden of chemical-laden fertilizers. Eating organic frees us from the disease-forming compounds that are used on so much of our modern food supply.

Eat the Rainbow of Colors and Reap the Medicinal Benefits

Fruits and vegetables in a variety of colors provide an abundance of vitamins, minerals, antioxidants, fiber, and *phytochemicals*— beneficial, nutrient-dense compounds found in plants—that the body uses to attain and maintain good health.

The five color categories are:

- Blue/purple
- Green
- White
- Yellow/orange
- Red

Each color has an extraordinary impact on maintaining optimal health and greatly reducing the risk of developing chronic diseases.

Blue/Purple helps lower our risk of some cancers, promotes urinary tract health, supports memory and concentration, maintains healthy kidney function, and supports healthy aging.

Green helps lower risk of some cancers, purifies the blood, promotes vision health, and supports strong bones and teeth.

White helps support a healthy immune system, maintain a lower risk of some cancers, leads to healthy cholesterol levels, and promotes heart health.

Yellow/Orange helps lower risk of some cancers, promotes heart and eye health, and supports a healthy immune system.

Red helps maintain a lower risk of some cancers, and aids in heart health, urinary tract health, and memory function.

You have probably noticed that all the colors in fruits and vegetables have potential anticancer benefits.

Nature's Fast Food

I encourage you to consume more fruits and vegetables each day. Plant-based foods are some of the most nutritionally dense foods on the planet. A diet rich in fruits and vegetables can lower blood pressure, reduce your risk of heart disease and stroke, prevent most types of cancers, and support healthy digestion. Eating more produce also has a positive effect upon blood glucose levels, which can help satisfy your appetite.

Diets high in fruits and vegetables are highly recommended for their health-promoting properties and provide exactly what we need to live the way God intended. Fruits and vegetables have an abundance of vitamins and minerals, especially vitamins C and A. They have extremely beneficial nutrients rich in anti-disease compounds.

Additionally, fruits and vegetables are recommended as an excellent source of dietary fiber. Fresh, organic produce, such as sliced apples, carrots, cherry tomatoes, avocados, diced peppers, and celery, serves as a quick and easy food to enjoy as healthy snacks or to curb a sugar craving. Next time you feel like a nibble or want to satisfy a craving, reach for one of these tasty, highly nutritious snacks instead of sugary, processed treats that pack on the pounds. Most cravings are caused by mineral deficiencies that lead to many health concerns, including weight gain.

The beneficial nutrients that fruits and vegetables provide play a critical role in health by protecting us against chronic diseases. So please, have a feast!

The Structure of Plants and Their Amazing Benefits

The structure of plants is where all the vital, ant disease nutrients are contained and therefore extremely necessary to obtain great health.

Fiber has many health benefits—most importantly, *healthy elimination* and a happy gut. Dietary fiber increases the weight and size of your stool and softens it. A heavier stool is easier to pass, decreasing your chance of constipation and *autointoxication* or self-poisoning. So, if you're having trouble moving your bowel, increase your fiber intake and get things moving.

Enzymes are necessary for digestion. When the Almighty Physician created fruit and vegetables, He filled them with all the necessary enzymes we need. For example, in juicy, sweet fruit there is *sucrose*, the enzyme required to digest sugar, *protease* for protein, *amylase* for carbohydrates, and *lipase* for digesting fat. Enzymes are catalysts that help us properly break down, assimilate, and metabolize our food.

Raw, lacto-fermented vegetables, like raw sauerkraut and kimchee, are cultured vegetables that contain beneficial probiotics and digestive enzymes. Lacto-fermentation is a method of food preservation that enhances the nutrient content in the food, making the nutrients, probiotics and enzymes more available and easier to digest. Consuming raw, lacto-fermented foods also restores friendly, or *good,* bacteria in our intestines, which reduce incidences of gas, bloating, constipation, and diarrhea. These good bacteria in fermented vegetables also have the ability to retard the growth of bad or unfriendly bacteria in the intestines, creating optimal immune function.

Flavonoids are found in almost every living plant. They construct the colors in the skins of fruits and vegetables. This nutrient group includes *anthocyanins, flavones, isoflavones, proantocyanidins, quercetin,* and more. For humans, flavonoids are potent antioxidants and help stop the growth of tumor cells. They also play a role in the reduction of inflammation.

Bioflavonoids, found in citrus fruits, are a compound related to vitamin C. This compound extends its value in the body when consumed. These nutrients have the ability to lower inflammatory levels and support joint collagen in arthritis and other inflammatory conditions.

Anthocyanins are antioxidant *flavonoids*. They protect many of our bodily systems. They have the strongest physiological effects of all plant species. Anthocyanins are chains of amino acid compounds. For plants, the colors attract pollinating insects and animals, ensuring that flowers develop into the fruit that will create more seeds. Anthocyanins also help protect plant leaves from ultraviolet radiation.

Quercetin: is the yellow pigment in citrus fruits that I like to call *the anti-allergen.* Not only does it help the body cope with allergens and other lung and breathing problems, but quercetin also works against accelerated aging and oxidative stress. Consume a variety of organic produce each day and look younger.

Chlorophyll: I like to call chlorophyll *the builder of blood.* The benefits include nourishment of our organ systems, prevention of anemia, and abundance of oxygen in the body. The pigment chlorophyll is what gives plant leaves their green color and for us humans, acts as a blood purifier. Chlorophyll is to plants what blood is to humans. It is the molecule in plants that absorbs and synthesizes sunlight into food energy in the process called *photosynthesis*.

Beta-glucan is found in mushrooms. It balances your body's immune system by supporting white blood cells. Beta-glucans have been shown to reduce the risk of many types of cancers. Beta-glucans boost the immune system and killer T-cell formation, which is our first line of defense against sickness and disease.

Ellagic Acid has been proven in many clinical studies to act as an antioxidant and anticarcinogen in the gastrointestinal tract. This nutrient also has been proven to have an antiproliferative effect on cancer cells. Ellagic acid is present in blueberries, raspberries, strawberries, pomegranates, and figs.

Beta-carotene, derived from the Latin *carota*, or carrot, is the orange or red plant pigment abundant in many plants and fruits — especially sweet potatoes, oranges, and mangos. Beta-carotene is a provitamin, which means its conversion into a vitamin (vitamin A in this case) occurs once we ingest it, especially when accompanied by a dietary fat.

Antioxidants are naturally occurring chemicals that can prevent or slow cell damage. An antioxidant is not an actual substance, but a behavior that inhibits oxidative stress or free radical damage. Any compound that can donate electrons and counteract free radicals has antioxidant properties. Antioxidants from fruits and vegetables benefit your body by neutralizing and removing from the bloodstream the free radicals that result in disease.

Phtyochemicals, also known as *phytonutrients*, are various bioactive chemical compounds found in plants. Antioxidants are considered to be beneficial to human health; phytochemicals are the compounds that make up antioxidants.

Polysaccharides are sugar units that can configure in long chains of tens to thousands of units. They comprise the carbohydrate storage component for plants and animals. Polysaccharides can also have structural roles in plants, fungi, and insects. *Homopolysaccharides* are starches and glycogen that have the same type of sugar throughout their chain.

Macronutrients are the structural and energy-giving caloric components of the foods we eat, including carbohydrates, fats, and proteins.

Micronutrients are the vitamins, minerals, trace elements, phytochemicals, and antioxidants that are essential for good health, including growth and development.

Carbohydrates are organic sugar compounds occurring in the fibers of fruits, vegetables, grains, starches, and milk products.

Simple carbohydrates are simple sugars that are made of one or two molecules of sugars. Simple carbohydrates break down quickly by the body to be used as energy. Some examples are fruits, honey, maple syrup, and milk products, such as yogurt, cheese, and kefir.

Complex carbohydrates are made up of sugar molecules that are bound together in long, complex chains and are found in foods, such as whole grains, legumes, and vegetables.

CHAPTER THREE

The Truth Will Set You Free

To obtain optimal health, we must go back to the way our ancestors ate and follow a traditional diet. You may be wondering what a *traditional diet* actually is. A traditional diet consists of foods that have not been altered from their original form. They contain all the necessary vitamins and minerals for optimal health. Traditional foods are always whole, unprocessed, and organic; free of chemical fertilizers and genetic mutations.

Organic Versus Nonorganic: Is There a Difference?

Have you ever wondered whether there is a difference between organic and nonorganic (conventional) and genetically engineered foods? Organic is the only way God intended for our food to be. The label "organic" generally means that foods have met a set of rigorous regional standards to be grown or prepared without synthetic additives, industrial solvents, artificial ingredients, or genetically modified foods. Organically grown foods can cost more, but you receive more value for your money. When you purchase nonorganic produce, you get up to 90 percent less nutritional value, along with all the dangerous, disease-forming compounds. It doesn't stop there; genetically modified organisms change the DNA of the produce, and chemical fertilizers are located in the cells of the produce. Neither can be washed off.

What Exactly Are Genetically Engineered Foods?

Genetic engineering alters the genetic makeup of an organism by inserting, deleting, or changing specific pieces of DNA. The manipulation of DNA is for the purpose of producing new types of organisms, usually by inserting or deleting genes with the use of bacteria. Genetic engineering has been developed commercially, with uses such as producing human insulin or bacteria.

Genetic manipulation of organisms includes splicing the genes from one species to another. It has been a source of controversy since the 1970s. Genetically engineered organisms are routinely used to create insulin and to produce biofuels. Corporate agriculture is heavily dependent on genetically engineered crops, such as corn and soybeans. It's frightening to say, but biotechnologists are creating what are essentially new species and even new kingdoms of life.

Dangers of GMOs

Genetically Modified Foods (GMOs) are foods that have been altered from their original form via gene splicing. For example, berries have a vulnerability to frost, which is why nature only allows them to grow successfully in warmer weather. Biotech giants, such as Monsanto, splice a gene from an unrelated species, such as an arctic flounder using bacteria, such as E. coli. These bacteria and genes are then injected into the seed of the berry. This process gives the berry the characteristics of the arctic flounder, which carries a natural antifreeze. The berry will now be able to grow year-round without a vulnerability to frost.

Although this may sound like a technological advancement of our food production, genetic engineering is doing the opposite by contributing to the ecological crisis in our soil and water supply.

Genetic engineering actually promotes crop failure because it makes crops more resistant to pesticides. Genetically modified foods are not recognized by the body. This results in autoimmune diseases, asthma, allergies, organ damage, infertility, intestinal bleeding, digestive disorders, and different types of cancers.

Genetically modified crops include rice, cotton, corn, sugar beets, canola, soybeans, peanuts, legumes, alfalfa, wheat, potatoes, and papaya.

Genetic engineering is a massive human experiment, and therefore the health risks are enormous. Genetically mutated organisms can be found in 80 percent of all processed foods in the United States.

Conventional Foods

Conventional foods are not genetically altered, but they do contain chemical fertilizers, pesticides, herbicides, and fungicides, all of which can accumulate in our organs and create disease. Purchasing organic foods will assure you of being free of GMOs and chemical additives that can greatly impact your health.

Monsanto, the Biotech Giant

Monsanto is a publicly traded American multinational, agrochemical, and agricultural biotechnology corporation headquartered in Creve Coeur, St. Louis, Missouri. It is a leading producer of genetically engineered (GE) seed and Roundup, a *glyphosate*-based herbicide. Glyphosate is a synthetic compound that is a genetically engineered herbicide typically used to destroy weeds. This herbicide has been known to cause serious skin irritation, allergies, asthma, and different types of cancers, such as lymphoma and leukemia.

Genetic engineering carries potential dangers:

- The creation of new allergens and toxins
- The evolution of new *super-weeds* and other noxious vegetation
- The harm of wildlife
- The creation of environments favorable to the proliferation of crops

Some scientists have expressed concern that new disease organisms and increased antibiotic resistance could result from the use of GMOs in the food chain.

Playing God

Genetic engineering (GE) is the deliberate manipulation of the genes in an organism with the intent of giving that organism the desired characteristics of an unrelated organism, as mentioned in the berry/flounder example. Inserting genes from unrelated species into plants and animals can cause existing genes to react in unknown ways, including reduced nutritional values and changes in organism quality.

When the resulting engineered plants resist insecticides, farmers find themselves having to spray more insecticide on the plants to achieve the same effect. Now triple that effect as pests build up insecticide resistance because of the larger usage of these toxoids, and you have a company selling more chemicals. The result is an environment that is more polluted, and a farmer growing increasingly dependent on the chemicals.

> *If my people, which are called by my name, shall humble themselves, and pray, and seek my face, and turn from their wicked ways; then will I hear from heaven, and will forgive their sin, and will heal their land.*
> —2 Chronicles 7:14 KJV

The Farmers Are Not to Blame

The reason to engineer and patent a seed is to make money. Although some family farmers in the United States may be using this technology, they are not the culprits. Genetically engineered crops lock farmers into a cycle of dependence on quick-fix schemes with royalty fees and debts to the bank. Farmers pay loyalty fees to save the seeds for the next year's crop. Quick-fix schemes supposedly protect the farmer from being sued by Monsanto, by exacting a fee from the farmer for the right to save the seeds.

Cross Contamination

The pollen from genetically engineered plants does not recognize buffer zones and containment fields. It drifts wherever the wind blows. Cross-contamination of conventional and nonorganic crops is a major concern for organic farming and the environment. These new creations have proven impossible to contain outside of a lab.

Who will be liable when this contamination occurs? Not the biotech companies. Currently there are few, if any, laws assigning liability to life's new architects. The laws that do exist are concerned with intellectual property rights. It seems the court wants to be certain you pay for every GE seed that grows, whether you planted it or not.

The World Produces More Than Enough Food

The promise to overcome worldwide hunger with the help of genetic engineering is not a solution, but a deception. Research and development of genetically modified plants are organized privately and lie in the hands of only a few big corporations. These corporations protect their products through patents.

Genetically modified plants do not contribute at all to the solution of agricultural problems; if anything, they contribute to the cause. Patents and technology fees prevent the transfer of technology. Lack of nutrition is not a problem of food quantity, but of power and distribution. The power is in the hands of the rich and powerful who keep the resources from the people. There is no scarcity of food anywhere in the world. The only scarcity is in the power to disconnect the people from their food.

The Myths Behind the Dirty Dozen and the Clean Fifteen

The concepts of *The Dirty Dozen* and *The Clean Fifteen* were designed to help consumers know when they should buy organic and when it is unnecessary. However, it is always necessary to free us of the toxic burden of chemical fertilizers that cannot be washed away. Remember, these chemicals are sprayed directly on the soil, from the time the crop is a seed until it's in full bloom, and are then located in the cells of the produce. This is exactly what we are feeding our families.

The lists below were compiled using data from the United States Department of Agriculture on the amount of pesticide residue found in nonorganic fruits and vegetables after they had been washed.

The Dirty Dozen, when conventionally grown, tested positive for at least forty-seven different chemicals, some testing positive for as many as sixty-seven. You should definitely buy organic of these foods unless you relish the idea of consuming a chemical cocktail.

The Dirty Dozen are sprayed with the most chemicals:

- Celery
- Peaches
- Strawberries
- Apples
- Domestic blueberries
- Nectarines
- Sweet bell peppers
- Spinach, kale, and collard greens
- Cherries
- Potatoes
- Imported grapes
- Lettuce

The list known as *The Clean Fifteen* are foods considered to have much lower pesticides on their crops.

All the produce on *The Clean Fifteen* have fewer chemical fertilizers and are a bit safer to consume in nonorganic form, in the event you cannot find these organic or need to budget your food shopping.

This list includes:

- Sweet corn
- Mango
- Onions
- Sweet peas
- Avocados
- Asparagus
- Kiwi fruit
- Cabbage
- Eggplant
- Cantaloupe
- Watermelon
- Grapefruit
- Sweet potatoes
- Sweet onions
- Pineapples

As long as any chemical fertilizers are being sprayed in any amount on produce, it can never be considered clean. Pesticides, fungicides, and other chemical-laden cocktails are sprayed on our produce, drenching the soil and plants from seeds to full bloom. These chemical compounds cannot be washed off because they are *inside* each cell of the produce. They do not belong on the menu.

Conventional farming practices see the soil as a moneymaking commodity, and their methods are driven by the almighty dollar. Soils are used and reused, and nutrients are drawn out of the soil by constantly growing the same crop in the same place. Without crop rotation, the soils are depleted. In the absence of naturally rich soil, farmers are forced to continue to saturate their crops with unnatural chemical fertilizers that destroy our food as well as our health.

These toxic chemical poisons that are sprayed on our food in any amount cause mineral deficiencies, such as the depletion of nitrogen, phosphorus, selenium, magnesium, and potassium, plus fifty additional important minerals that are needed to nourish our produce. One sample of conventional produce tested with thirty-three pesticide residues, of which five are neurotoxins, fifteen disrupt hormones, thirteen are carcinogens, and all have the potential to cause allergies and asthma.

Washing Won't Take It Away!

Poor soil health leads to poor plant health. When plants are deficient, they lose their defenses against pests, and diseases come. Once this nightmare occurs, the farmers go crying to the big chemical companies for help. These big poison conglomerates are more than happy to supply deadly toxins like pesticides, herbicides, and fungicides.

Conventional farming yields not just poor soil and plant health, but also a deficient and toxic food supply, which lead to our bodies becoming deficient and toxic.

Age is not a prerequisite to disease.

Keep in mind that these chemical concoctions cause vitamin and mineral deficiencies that manifest in us as mood swings, lack of energy, joint pain, failing eyesight, and hearing loss. The deficiencies contribute to major illnesses, such as cancer, heart disease, diabetes, mental illness, allergies, asthma, infertility, digestive issues, hormonal problems, and thousands of other ailments that medical science would tell us to accept as a normal case of aging. Monsanto and other biotech companies claim GMOs have no impact on the environment and are perfectly safe to eat. Imagine!

Price Look Up (PLU) Number

When purchasing produce, you must look at the Price Look Up or PLU numbers. PLU numbers are the stickers on each item that describe with a four- or five-digit number whether the product is organic, nonorganic, or GMO. For example, organic produce has a five-digit PLU code beginning with the number 9. Conventionally or pesticide-grown produce has a 4-digit PLU code, and begins with the number 4, genetically modified produce has a 5-digit PLU code beginning with the number 8.

Remember: purchasing produce with the PLU beginning with the number 9 will assure you that your produce is organic.

Here are two simple principals to avoid genetically modified foods:

1. Avoid pre-packed and processed foods.
2. Look for the USDA Organic seal.

Here is a list of fruits and vegetables that should be consumed generously.

Vegetables (preferably organic)

- Artichokes
- Arugula
- Asparagus
- Beets
- Broccoli
- Broccoli rabe
- Brussels sprouts
- Cabbage
- Carrots
- Cauliflower

- Celery
- Collard greens
- Corn
- Cucumber
- Dandelion
- Eggplant
- Endive
- Escarole
- Garlic
- Kale
- Lettuce of all varieties
- Mushrooms
- Mustard greens
- Okra
- Onion
- Peas
- Peppers
- Pumpkin
- Radicchio
- Raw, lacto-fermented sauerkraut and other fermented vegetables
- Romaine
- Sea vegetables: dulse, nori, kombu, kelp
- Spinach
- Sprouts: alfalfa, broccoli, sunflower, pea shoots, and radish
- Squash, winter or summer
- String beans
- Sweet potatoes
- Tomatoes
- Yams
- Zucchini

Fruits (preferably organic)

- Apples
- Apricots
- Banana
- Blackberries
- Blueberries
- Cherries
- Cranberries
- Dried fruit, with no added sulphites or sugar: raisins, figs, dates, prunes, pineapple, papaya
- Grapes
- Grapefruit
- Guava
- Kiwi
- Lemon
- Lime
- Mango
- Melon
- Mulberries
- Oranges
- Papaya
- Passion fruit
- Peaches
- Pears
- Pineapple
- Plums
- Pomegranates
- Raspberries
- Strawberries

Eating in Season

Seasonal food is significantly more delicious and nutritious than food grown out of season. Foods that have had the chance to fully and naturally ripen before they've been picked will taste exactly how they are supposed to. Have you ever eaten a fully ripe tomato in the summer and enjoyed how sweet and refreshing it is, as opposed to a tomato in midwinter?

Studies have shown that produce grown in season and under appropriate conditions has up to three times more nutrients than those grown out of season. Local fruits and vegetables don't have to endure as much travel, so they don't lose those vital nutrients. Eating local foods in season supports small farmers as well as your local community.

Eating in season is not only healthier, but it can also be less expensive since you're not paying for transport. When you buy what's in season, you buy food that's at the peak of its supply, and it costs less to farmers who harvest and transport it to your grocery stores or farmers' markets. It may seem like common sense to buy locally grown and in season, but it's one of those things many of us ignore when shopping.

This link can help you find what's in season around you: sustainabletable.org/seasonalfoodguide.

Here is a general list of what's in season in the Northeast:

January: cabbage, cauliflower, rhubarb, leeks, parsnips, turnip, shallots, squash

February: cabbage, cauliflower, celeriac, chard, chicory, leeks, parsnips, spinach, swede, turnip

March: beetroot, cabbage, cauliflower, leeks, mint, parsley, broccoli, radishes, rhubarb

April: broccoli, cabbage, cauliflower, morel mushrooms, wild garlic, radishes, rhubarb, carrots, kale, watercress, spinach

May: broccoli, cabbage, cauliflower, gooseberries, parsley, mint, broad beans, rhubarb, new carrots, asparagus

June: carrots, cherries, elderflowers, lettuce, strawberries, peppers, asparagus, red currants, peas, rhubarb, gooseberries, tomatoes, courgettes (zucchini), broad beans

July: carrots, gooseberries, strawberries, spinach, tomatoes, watercress, loganberries, sage, cauliflower, aubergine (eggplant), fennel, asparagus, cabbage, celery, cherries, lettuce, mangetout (snowpeas), nectarines, new potatoes, oyster mushrooms, peas, peaches, radish, raspberries, rhubarb, tomatoes, french beans

August: carrots, gooseberries, lettuce, raspberries, strawberries, cauliflower, aubergines, nectarines, peaches, peppers, courgettes, rhubarb, sweet corn, basil, peas, pears, apples, french beans, tomatoes

September: apples, aubergines, blackberries, cabbage, carrots, cauliflower, cucumber, damsons, elderberries, figs, french beans, grapes, kale, lettuce, melons, mushrooms, nectarines, onions, peppers, parsnips, peas, peaches, pears, potatoes, pumpkin, raspberries, rhubarb, spinach, sweet corn, tomatoes

October: apples, aubergines, beetroot, cabbage, carrots, cauliflower, courgettes, grapes, lettuce, marrow (gourd), mushrooms, parsnips, potatoes, squash, tomatoes, watercress

November: cabbage, pumpkin, swede, cauliflower, potatoes, parsnips, pears, leeks, quinces, chestnuts, cranberries, beetroot

December: celery, cabbage, red cabbage, cauliflower, celeriac, clementines, pumpkin, beetroot, turnips, parsnips, satsumas, sprouts, pears, pomegranate, swede

CHAPTER FOUR

Your Eggs May Not Be All That They Are Cracked Up To Be

Organic Eggs

The incredible, edible egg is here at last! Now don't get too excited, because organic eggs and chickens are not automatically the best choice. Chickens can be labeled as organically raised when they are given organic feed, but they may very well be in a factory-like setting. Organically raised hens might not consume nature's salad bar of flora and fauna that deliver optimum health and happiness. Keep in mind that chickens consuming grain and only grain, organic or not, produce eggs that are too high in omega-6 fatty acids and contain almost no omega-3s.

Omega-3s are called *good fats* because they play a critical role in every cell in your body. Omegas-3s are formed in the chloroplast of green leaves from natural forage.

People who have diets with sufficient amounts of omega-3s are less likely to have high blood pressure, arthritis, and other inflammatory conditions. Omega-3s are essential for your brain and neurological health as well. People with a diet rich in omega-3s are also less likely to suffer from depression, attention deficit disorder, and Alzheimer's disease.

Vegetarian Fed

Now keep in mind that chickens are not vegetarians. They are omnivores, which means they eat from both animal and plant kingdoms. Chickens feast on insects, frogs, worms, and plants; they are not just plant eaters.

The Color of Egg Shells

Many people ask me if they purchase brown eggs are they getting a better quality egg. The color of the shell has absolutely nothing to do with the nutritional value of the egg or how the hen is fed. Chicken eggs come in all colors including shades of brown, white, blue, olive, and rose, depending on the breed of the chicken. Ameraucana hens produce light blue, white, and even pale pink eggs. Despite the color of the shell, if the hens are poorly fed or inhumanely raised, their nutritional content is automatically lessened, as well as their quality.

Pasture-Raised or Free-Roaming Eggs

Pasture-raised eggs are the way to go. Yes, here's to a healthy omelet! Pastured hens freely roam outdoors where they can forage for their natural diet, including seeds, green plants, insects, and worms. Pasture-raised eggs are extremely high in omega-3s (for more about omega-3s and good fats, see chapter ten). Additionally, the freely roaming chicken's diet is rich in iron, zinc, calcium, magnesium, conjugated linoleic acid (CLA), and vitamin E. Pasture-raised chickens are not fed antibiotics, corn, or soy.

Nutrients virtually disappear when the hens feast on an abundance of grain and lack forage. One way to assess the nutrient level of the laying hens is to observe the color of the egg yolk. Pastured hens produce eggs with deep orange yolks. Pale yellow yolks are a major indicator that you're getting eggs from caged hens.

Typically, if you live in an urban area, visiting a local health food store would be your best route to finding the highest quality eggs. Your local farmers' market may be another source for pasture-raised hens and their eggs.

Get to know your food and your farmer. You should visit the farms your eggs have come from. I enjoy going to farms; it's educational and a wonderful way to connect with nature and your food source. Don't be afraid to ask questions about what the chickens you are eating have eaten or their living conditions. Farmers are generally happy to show off their methods, as long as they've got nothing to hide. Your egg farmer should be loyal to the hens' diet, water source, and plenty of open roaming space to reduce stress on the hens and support their immune systems. Interestingly, we are not only what we eat, but also what our food is eating.

To sum up, you want your chicken and eggs to be certified organic *and* pasture-raised.

Storage

Please note that fresh, pastured-raised eggs from happy, healthy hens can be stored without refrigeration for up to two weeks. This is well-known in many other countries, including parts of Europe. Here in the United States, organic farmers often do not refrigerate their eggs. The shelf life of a healthy, unrefrigerated egg is approximately seven to fourteen days, compared to most factory eggs that are refrigerated for up to fifty days. Keep this in mind when purchasing eggs from a grocery store. By the time they hit the refrigerated shelves, they may already be four to six weeks old. Once again, my suggestion is to purchase your eggs from a local, pastured source.

Does Eating Eggs Cause Heart Disease?

While it's true that fats from animal sources contain cholesterol, I promise you this is not necessarily something that will harm you. Eggs from the right source can be one of the healthiest foods you can eat. Pastured eggs may help prevent heart disease since they are extremely high in heart-healthy nutrients, including omega-3s, CLA, vitamin E, and magnesium—four necessary nutrients for a healthy heart.

One 2009 study discovered that the proteins in cooked eggs are converted by gastrointestinal enzymes, producing peptides that act as ACE inhibitors—Angiotensin-converting-enzyme inhibitor is a pharmaceutical drug used primarily for the treatment of hypertension (high blood pressure) and CHF (congestive heart failure). Although egg yolks are high in cholesterol, there are numerous studies that have confirmed that eggs do not raise your blood serum cholesterol levels.

Here's why blaming dietary cholesterol for heart disease is like blaming the police for the crime: elevated cholesterol levels are an indication that your body is under attack from a highly inflammatory diet. Your brain sends signals to your liver, the manufacturer of the antioxidant cholesterol, to send more of it when the body is in trouble and in need of repair.

Cholesterol is a repair substance and is not correlated with heart disease. It is highly beneficial in the production of hormones, especially the feel-good hormones known as *serotonin*, *oxytocin*, and *dopamine*. Cholesterol is also essential for a healthy brain. Patients taking cholesterol-lowering drugs known as *statins* have complained of memory loss and concentration issues. I have had many new patients taking statins and they are also on antidepressants due to the happy-hormone depletion from these drugs.

I consider cholesterol my friend, not my enemy.

Now, I would love to invite you over for my delicious egg recipe but instead, I encourage you to make it yourself.

Tonijean's Olde World Frittata

Preheat oven to 350°F.

Ingredients:
Extra virgin coconut oil
6 pastured eggs
1 cup fresh or frozen organic vegetables, chopped
¼ to ½ cup of your favorite raw organic cheese, grated
Celtic or unrefined salt
Black pepper
Organic powdered garlic
Organic powdered onion

Grease the bottom of baking dish with coconut oil.

Beat the eggs in a separate bowl and pour into the baking dish.

Add veggies of choice. I like to use broccoli florets, chopped zucchini, onion, and garlic, but any veggies will do.

Then season with salt and pepper to taste and a few pinches of powdered garlic and onion.

Sprinkle shredded cheese evenly on the top.

Bake for about twenty-five minutes. Remove when fully cooked, when a knife inserted into the center comes out clean and the cheese is bubbly and browned at the edges.

Cut into triangles or squares.

Serve this easy, delicious, and nutritious meal any time of the day. I like to eat this with a mixed green salad.

Factory-Farmed Poultry

Sadly, factory-farmed poultry are crowded in dark rooms, unable to see the light of day. These beautiful creatures have the pointed tips of their beaks cut off to reduce the excessive feather pecking and cannibalism seen within these stressed, overcrowded conditions. These birds become your typical supermarket chicken or turkey. These battery-raised chickens never have a chance to scratch, eat worms, bugs, and natural forage. The name battery-raised was coined from the arrangement of columns of identical cages connected together, similar to common divider walls of the cells in a battery.

Mother hens are separated from their chicks immediately after hatching. Despite the cruel separation, baby chicks are able to identify their mother hen by various communication strategies, and hearing seems to be an important one. When a sitting hen was removed in the dark from her chicks and another broody hen put in her place, the chicks still found their own mother hen. Although the hen was crammed with hundreds of hens and disguised by inhumane conditions, her chicks came to her anyway. That to me is the precious gift that only nature can provide. This wonderful means of communication is taken away from them through the horror of the mass chicken-egg production industry.

Chickens and all living creatures have the ability to love and feel pain, both physically and emotionally.

More than 85 percent of store-bought and restaurant chickens are now factory-farmed. The mass production of eggs often creates unsanitary conditions and causes recalls due to salmonella. The poisonous and infectious bacterial diseases can all be avoided by practicing proper, humane farming methods.

I'm sure an omelet is not sounding too appealing right now.

The life of any animal is not any less precious than that of a human being.

CHAPTER FIVE

The Dark Side of the Meat and Dairy Industry

There is little that separates humans from other sentient beings. We all feel joy, we all crave to be alive and to live freely, and we all share this planet together.

—Mahatma Gandhi

You Are What *They* Eat

I choose to be a vegetarian, but for those who choose to consume meat, there are many considerations I write about in this chapter. The meat, poultry, and dairy foods consumed by our ancestors were much different than what we eat today. Livestock was treated humanely, without the use of growth hormones and antibiotics. Dairy, meats, and eggs were packed with beneficial enzymes and the proper ratio of omega-3 and omega-6 fatty acids. The livestock feasted on wild legumes, natural forage, and rapidly growing grass while enjoying abundant sunlight and fresh air.

Inhumane animal cruelty, called *factory farming*, is one of the toughest topics that I have ever had to learn and teach. I can honestly say this is the most difficult section for me as I write this book. Although the Bible does speak clearly of meat and dairy as being healthy for our consumption, factory farming was certainly not part of the equation. What follows is a graphic, albeit accurate, depiction of the practices taking place within the meat and dairy industry to produce that all-American dinner on your plate.

The problem with factory farms is that they don't produce healthy, safe food, or a clean environment. The livestock are overcrowded with tens of thousands of animals crammed into dark factories where they never see the light of day, which interrupts the animal's natural circadian rhythm. In other cases, the factories are lit with fluorescents that are never turned off, and therefore the animals are in permanent daylight, which is considered a torture/interrogation tactic in humans. With this horror also come millions of tons of manure, water pollution, air pollution, and dangerous conditions for those living nearby.

The growth of factory farms in recent decades is destroying the small and medium-scale livestock farms that can provide good food for us and good economies for communities.

Even if you aren't living near a factory farm, you aren't immune from the problems they cause. Illness from factory-farmed food products, such as outbreaks of food poisoning and even death, has occurred due to salmonella and E. coli. Many factory farm operators don't benefit from this system of production due to the lack of adequate compensation for the mistreated livestock they raise.

Some of the detrimental effects of factory farming are:

- Animal welfare problems
- Environmental issues
- Ecological devastation
- Public health endangerment
- Food safety risks
- Economic loss

Factory farming effects also include dangerous conditions and low pay scales for human workers. No one benefits except the one making money from all the abuse. The rise of factory farming has resulted from public policy choices driven by big agribusinesses. The processors of the meat and meat packers also control the steps taken between factory farming and the consumer. Don't be deceived by the beautiful green, plush meadows portrayed in advertising. Most of the pork, beef, poultry, dairy, and eggs produced in the United States (land of the free), come from large-scale and confined factory farms.

Factory farm livestock operations also create public health hazards in other ways. When thousands of beef cattle are packed into feedlots full of manure, bacteria can get on their hides and then into the slaughterhouses where your food is produced. Contamination on even one steer can contaminate thousands of pounds of meat inside a slaughterhouse, contributing to E. coli and other disease-forming compounds in your store-bought USDA choice cuts. Now you don't have wonder where mad cow disease came from.

The facilities are overcrowded and extremely stressful to animals, making it easy for disease to spread. These poor animals are too weak and sick to walk onto the planks heading for slaughter. The USDA will allow the sickest, weakest animals to be ground up as feed used for cattle food. I hope you now look a bit differently at your ground beef patties.

These industrial operations are all about mass production for profit and nothing else. Animal factories house thousands of animals raised for profit, such as chickens, turkeys, cows, and pigs. Due to these crammed, overcrowded conditions, they are treated with hormones and antibiotics to prevent disease and maximize their growth, again, strictly for profit. Animals are fed genetically engineered corn and soy that are grown through intensive industrial farming methods using large amounts of pesticides, herbicides, and chemical fertilizers. These poisons remain in the animals' bodies and are passed on to the people who eat them, creating serious health hazards in humans.

> *Our task must be to free ourselves . . . by widening our circle of compassion to embrace all living creatures and the whole of nature and its beauty.*
>
> — Albert Einstein

From Calf to Feedlot to Your Dinner Table

Now that you are learning about the horror of mass beef production in the United States, allow me to elaborate. Most beef cattle are born on independent farms somewhere in the West. On a healthy farm, they would normally spend the first six months on real pasture with their mothers, enjoying a salad bar of real grass and forage that nature designed for their diet. Unfortunately, in the beef production industry, this type of farm is called a *cow-calf operation*. It is called an operation because the calf wasn't conceived the way nature intended. The calf was the product of artificial insemination. Babies are taken from their mother while crying out of fear and separation and moved to a dark pen. The mother suffers no differently than a human mother losing her baby. Cows have the same exact feelings and nurturing aspects as do we humans. The calf will spend the next couple months in the feedlot eating from a trough and being given genetically modified corn and soy, growing to as much as six hundred pounds. Then the calf will be branded and, if male, castrated as the cattle farmers prep them for future meals sent to local supermarkets and butcher shops for your food.

Factory-Farmed Milk Production

As an animal lover, it is extremely difficult to write about the cruel horror of factory farming. However, I believe it is extremely important for you to be aware. Did you know that cows form lifelong friendships, for instance? They play games with one another, have emotions, and possess distinct personality traits.

Unfortunately, in today's modern milking industry, cows do not have the opportunity to live happily ever after. Female cows are deprived of nursing their calves, the way nature intended, even for a day. After they give birth, the baby is removed immediately from the mother while she remains in emotional pain and suffering.

Cows are treated like milk-producing machines and are genetically manipulated, pumped full of antibiotics and growth hormones that cause them to produce astronomical amounts of milk. *Mastitis*, a painful, pus-filled infection of the mammary glands, is much more likely to develop from this massive milk production. These infectious secretions flow into the milk supply and are sent to supermarkets for us to drink. While these cows suffer on factory farms, humans who drink the milk from this source increase their chances of developing many different diseases.

Oh, did I tell you that the USDA allows for blood and pus to enter our milk supply? Don't worry, though; they use bleaching agents as disinfectants and whiteners to hide the color variations from you. Doesn't that make you feel better?

Detrimental Effects of Hormones in Your Food

Hormones injected into your food supply mimic or interfere with the function of hormones within your body. Your endocrine system becomes overloaded and confused, which affects the normal functions of tissues and organs.

Many of these substances have been linked with imbalances in normal hormonal function, resulting in a variety of diseases:

- Estrogen-dominant cancers
- Developmental issues
- Reproduction issues
- Early menstruation
- Early menopause
- Infertility
- Heart disease due to elevated homocysteine levels
- Gynecomastia, or enlarged breasts in boys and men
- Hair loss
- Obesity
- Diabetes

The female cows are artificially inseminated shortly after they are a year old. After giving birth, they lactate for ten months and are then inseminated again, and again, continuing the massive production. Some cows spend their entire lives standing on concrete floors while others are confined to massive, crowded crates where they are forced to stand and live in their own feces. Healthy cows in general have a natural lifespan of about twenty years and can produce milk for eight or nine years. However, the stress caused by these factory conditions can only lead to disease, which shortens their lifespans.

Unfortunately, many of these poor cows develop reproductive issues due to this horrific farming method and are then considered by the dairy industry to be worthless. Now, keep in mind that they are only about four years of age at this point, but they are sent to be slaughtered for your burgers and steaks since they are too sick to produce milk.

Pasteurized Dairy, Bone Loss, and Heart Disease

All the vital nutrients, including calcium, are boiled to death through the pasteurization process. Consuming pasteurized dairy products contributes to bone thinning (*osteopenia*) and bone loss (*osteoporosis*). This process is due to the calcium leaching from your bones, traveling into your blood, and then creating what's known as *hardening of the arteries*. The physiology of pasteurized milk is destroyed, making it a highly acidic and unhealthy food. The biggest storage of calcium in the body is in the bones, and if the calcium in milk is destroyed through pasteurization, the calcium of the consumer will also be destroyed. Oxidation of the fat and cholesterol also occur, which are even greater offenses for heart disease and bone loss.

At this point you're probably wondering why pasteurization was necessary. This process was not for your safety, but so the farmer can practice inhumane, unsanitary farming methods that allowed the farmer to rapidly produce lots of milk for profit. The end result is a lot of milk with much less quality and a ton of disease-forming pathogens.

Now keep in mind, not all farmers use pasteurization as a method to treat animals inhumanely for profit. There are many honest farmers who pasteurize as a means of safety and to obey the law. Pasteurization dramatically reduced the incidence of illnesses like tuberculosis, although the process kills helpful bacteria as well as pathogens, and leaves behind a far less nutritious product.

There are many small farmers who raise cows ethically, kindly, and humanely, yet pasteurize the milk in order to sell it to a larger vendor. They do not pasteurize to be inhumane, but because they believe they are creating a healthier, more marketable product.

Pasteurization also extends the shelf life of milk. There is a process called *ultra pasteurization,* in which the milk is heated a second time. The expiration date on ultra-pasteurized milk is now extended to two months. Your safety was the original reason why pasteurization was first developed; however, some big farm corporations use pasteurization strictly to extend shelf life and gain profit.

Remember, when you purchase food with a longer shelf life, the shorter the quality of life of the consumer.

The Evil Production of Pork

It is difficult to say which factory-farmed animals are treated most inhumanely; however, I would say pigs are probably the highest ranking in abuse. Pigs are sweet and intelligent animals, yet are probably the most mistreated for food profit in factory farming. Please prepare yourself as you continue to read this mass horror that most consider food.

Mother pigs, who number almost seven million in the United States, spend most of their lives in individual gestation crates. These crates are about seven feet long and two feet wide, making them too small to allow the animals to turn around, let alone walk. After giving birth to their piglets, they are moved to farrowing crates, which are not wide enough for them to lie down and nurse their babies. These crates are not big enough for them to turn around or build secure bedding for their young as they were created to do.

The babies are then separated from their mothers when they are as young as ten days old. Once her piglets are gone, the mother pig is impregnated again, like a machine, and the cycle continues for three or four years until she is slaughtered for food. At this point, she is just too sick to handle reproduction.

After they are taken from their mothers, baby piglets are confined to small pens until they are ready to be raised for meat. Every year in the United States, millions of male piglets are castrated without pain killers due to consumers supposedly complain of *boar taint*, an offensive odor and taste that can be evident in the meat of this barbaric industry. Another reason for castration is to lower testosterone and make it easier to take full control of the pig. Piglets are not exposed to this abuse in some European countries; it is mostly here in the land of the free that this practice takes place.

In these extremely crowded conditions, piglets are prone to stress-related behavior, such as cannibalism and tail biting, because they go insane from the massive abuse. Factory farmers often chop off piglets' tails and use pliers to break off the ends of their teeth—once again—without giving them anything for the horrendous pain. To top it off, factory farmers also cut off parts of the pig's ears for identification purposes.

A typical slaughterhouse kills about one thousand hogs per hour. The number of animals killed makes it impossible for pigs' deaths to be painless. An electrical device known as a stun gun is used to stun or shock the pig before slaughter. The sensation is similar to being electrocuted. Because of improper stunning, many pigs are found squealing from the torment and severe pain. Inspectors found hogs that were walking and squealing after being stunned as many as six times. After the horrific death, pigs' hair is removed before butchering by submerging them in scalding-hot water baths that soften their skin and make the hair easier to remove. Some pigs are still alive when they reach the baths.

I am in love with nature and animals. Writing this section of my book is upsetting and painful, as I am sure it is for you to read it. I do believe, however, that it is necessary for everyone to know exactly where their food comes from.

For those who choose to eat meat, they have the right to know of the unfair, inhumane, cruel, and unnecessary methods of meat production.

I hope you now look at your omelets, pork chops, beef patties, Thanksgiving turkey, and roasted chicken dinner quite differently.

You Become What They Endure

When you think it can't get any worse than this, think again.

The same exact emotions of fear, sadness, anxiety, and pain that the animal endured is present in their body. When their flesh is turned into a food product, those emotions are still present. When one partakes in any factory-farmed product, one is taking in those same emotions. Slaughtered, abused animals become a part of our emotions when we consume the products made from these hopeless, inhumanely raised creatures.

> *If a man aspires toward a righteous life, his first act of abstinence is from injury to animals.*
> — Albert Einstein

Factory-Farmed Sheep and Lamb

Sheep and lambs have great memories and are super-intelligent, precious animals. They remember the animals and humans that they have met, and form lasting friendships with their flocks. Some neuroscientists now believe that the sheep's brain recognizes faces in the same way a human does.

In nature, sheep have the exact compassion as do humans in close-knit families. Each flock stays together, and the members of the flock protect each other. How beautiful is that? As they wander, one sheep ventures ahead of the group as a lookout for the others. A second sheep follows, and then signals to the rest of the herd that it is safe to come along. Sheep are like an army of protective soldiers looking after one another.

Sheep and lambs appear to form individual friendships, grazing consistently with the same companions. Like humans, sheep think about their friends even when they are not together. They also become worried and stressed when their companions are missing from the flock.

The Wool Over Your Eyes

It's horrific what these amazing and beautiful animals go through for mass profit. In the inhumane, money-driven industry, sheep are bred to produce unnaturally high quantities of wool. Sheep naturally grow just enough wool to protect themselves from frigid temperatures. Sheepshearing is the process in which the wool is cut off. The process of shearing can be extremely stressful for sheep and quite traumatic. The combination of forceful restraint, along with the pressure and heat from shears, causes a rapid elevation in *cortisol levels*, a primary factor of fear in both humans and animals.

Additionally, shearers are usually paid by volume, not by the hour, which leads to quick work without any regard for the welfare of the sheep. Shear sheds or wool sheds are large sheds that accommodate sheepshearing. These facilities are one of the worst places in the world for cruelty to animals. The workers of this cruel industry have literally punched sheep to subdue them with their shears or their fists until the sheep's nose bleeds.

There are many practices adopted by factory farms, or farmers trying to increase their yields, in the name of convenience and efficiency. If there were fewer animals on the farm or if the farmers had more time, likely these practices would be abandoned and deemed unnecessary. But money drives the market, and the more products the farmer can deliver, the more money they can pocket.

In many cases, this process causes them to override compassion and common sense regarding how to treat another living being.

Some of the practices for raising sheep are geared toward reducing the risk of fly-strike, in which flies lay eggs in feces that is stuck to the animal's hindquarters. The larva can then enter the sheep's body and cause a painful death. Industrial farmers have attempted to solve this problem with a variety of cheap, cruel methods, including tail docking.

Over 90 percent of U.S. lambs have their tails docked or cut off within the first few days of life. The idea is that this will prevent infection of bacteria and flies by keeping their vents or anuses clear of obstruction. In extreme cases, these helpless animals can suffer rectal prolapse, in which the tail muscles weaken and force the rectum to painfully protrude from the anus.

Merino sheep have more wrinkly skin and are more prone to fly strike, so they undergo a terrifying practice called *mulesing*. Not only the tail, but also large pieces of skin covering the buttocks are then sliced off, without any painkillers. This cruel and evil act leads to smooth scar tissue that won't retain moisture and attract flies. The alternative would be to sanitize the sheep's rear with a clean cloth every few months, but imagine, this isn't considered worth the labor cost.

Another painful mutilation includes dehorning, whereby the sensitive horn buds are seared off with a hot iron, preventing the growth of horns as the animal matures.

Young rams are castrated by the placement of a tight elastic ring around the male sheep's testicles until they fall off.

Did I mention that these practices are all done *without* any painkillers? At this point, you are probably wondering why and how all these cruel and evil acts could actually exist.

Slaughtering Practices

Another source of income from sheep is meat production. Please be aware, the content in this section is quite disturbing and extremely upsetting for me to write, as well as it will be for you to read and learn how lamb is produced in the factory-farmed industry. Lamb is the term for the meat that comes from sheep younger than a year old. Mutton is the name of the meat from sheep that are older than one year. Mutton has a stronger, gamier flavor. Lambs are slaughtered between the ages of two months and ten months old in inhumane cruelty.

When lamb and sheep arrive at commercial slaughtering facilities, they are unloaded, weighed, and placed in a restraining chute. They are treated as if they are objects, not living things. Before being slaughtered, each animal is supposed to be rendered unconscious. The goal is to penetrate the brain but not sever the brain stem. If the brain stem is severed, then the heart would stop pumping blood and the animal would not bleed out as quickly or completely as desired. The tool that is used for this horrific procedure is a captive bolt pistol.

The pistol is placed tightly against the animal's forehead and a long, pointed bolt is shot into the brain, causing the animal to spasm uncontrollably and then collapse. After being shackled by a hind leg and raised off the ground, the sheep is cut from the stomach to the throat and left to bleed. The animals sometimes regain consciousness due to improper stunning and have their throats slit, or dismantled, while totally aware. This is done, once again, without any pain medications.

I realize how difficult it has been for you to read this segment of my book. However, as a consumer, I do believe it is your right and responsibility to know exactly what your family may be eating, or where the fiber they wear comes from—and how these poor victims are mistreated in this horrible industry. You now know that you do have the choice in choosing humanely treated meats for yourself and your loved ones, as well as the welfare of livestock.

> *The more helpless the creature, the more that it is entitled to protection by man from the cruelty of man.*
> —Mahatma Gandhi

CHAPTER SIX

Humane Farming Practices

Now that you have a general idea of the dark side of the meat and dairy industry, let me explain the brighter side of humane, happy, healthy livestock.

As you know by now, I base my nutrition information on the principles stated clearly in biblical scripture. Let's begin by reviewing the scriptures on clean and unclean meats.

As representatives of Christ, the Almighty Physician, we will have fewer incidences of cancer, heart disease, digestive issues, brain and neurological disorders, and so on, I believe, simply because we follow guidelines and principles stated clearly in scripture. We will shine with radiant health, so the rest of the world will want what we have. This is called *ministering with our bodies*.

> *Therefore, I urge you, brothers and sisters, in view of God's mercy, to offer your bodies as a living sacrifice, holy and pleasing to God — this is your true and proper worship.*
> — Romans 12:1 NIV

When it pertains to meat, the Bible doesn't actually say that we will *burn in hell* if we eat pork or crustaceans. However, crustaceans are bottom feeders, the vacuum cleaners of the ocean. Shrimp, lobster, clams, and all shellfish are the cleaners of the oceans; what they eat becomes their flesh.

The diet of pigs naturally includes leaves, roots, insects, fruits, and even small animals. They are omnivores and indiscriminate. They will eat many things other animals will pass by. On the farm, pigs are often used as scavengers. Their handlers often feed them waste. In the overcrowded, cramped conditions of a factory farm, they will eat their own feces, as well as the carcasses of sick animals, including their own young. In a natural, healthy environment, pigs do not eat their own feces. They are fastidious by nature. In a pen with adequate space, they pee and poop in one corner, not indiscriminately like horses, sheep, and cows.

This may explain why the meat of the pig can be considered unclean or at least not so appetizing to consume. A pig digests whatever it eats quickly; they have only one stomach. A cow, with four stomachs, takes twenty-four hours to digest what it has eaten. During the digestive process, animals get rid of excess toxins, as well as other components of the food eaten that could be dangerous to health. Since the pig's digestive system operates rather basically, many of these toxins remain in their system to be stored in their more-than-adequate fatty tissues, ready for our consumption.

Another major issue regarding the buildup of toxins in pork is that pigs don't have any sweat glands. Sweat glands are another outlet the body uses to expel toxins. This leaves more toxins in the pig's body; and therefore, parasites are highly likely. Yes,

I am referring to both pastured-fed, humanely raised pork as well as factory-farmed, inhumanely treated pigs.

> *And the Lord spoke to Moses and Aaron, saying to them, "Speak to the people of Israel, saying, these are the living things that you may eat among all the animals that are on the earth. Whatever parts the hoof and is cloven-footed and chews the cud, among the animals, you may eat. Nevertheless, among those that chew the cud or part the hoof, you shall not eat these: The camel, because it chews the cud but does not part the hoof, is unclean to you. And the rock badger, because it chews the cud but does not part the hoof, is unclean to you.*
> — Leviticus 11:1-5 ESV

God states that cud-chewing animals with cloven or split hooves can be eaten (Leviticus: 11:3).

(Deuteronomy: 14:6) These specifically include the cattle, sheep, goat, deer, and gazelle families (Deuteronomy: 14:4–5).

He also lists such animals as camels, rabbits, and pigs as being unclean, or unfit to eat (Leviticus: 11:4-8).

He later lists such "creeping things" as moles, mice, and lizards as unfit to eat (Leviticus: 11:29–31), as well as four-footed animals with paws (cats, dogs, bears, lions, tigers, etc.) as unclean (Leviticus: 11:27).

He tells us that salt and freshwater fish with fins and scales may be eaten (Leviticus: 11:9–12), but water creatures without those characteristics (catfish, lobsters, crabs, shrimp, mussels, clams, oysters, squid, and octopi) should not be eaten.

God also lists birds and other flying creatures that are unclean for consumption (Leviticus: 11:13:19). He identifies carrion eaters and birds of prey as unclean, plus ostriches, storks, herons, and bats.

Birds, such as chickens, turkeys, and pheasants, are not on the unclean list and therefore, can be eaten. Insects, with the exception of locusts, crickets, and grasshoppers, are listed as unclean (Leviticus: 11:23).

Organic Meats and Eggs Versus Grass-fed and Pasture-Raised

Organic meats and eggs are a step in a better direction, however, that is better than factory-farmed food sources. Organically fed animals may still be in confinement while given organic grains. Cows do not have the ability to digest grain, making them susceptible to digestive disorders that lead to disease. Again, remember the ratio of omega-3 to omega-6. Farm animals are healthiest when they graze on nature's salad bar.

As mentioned in chapter four, when these animals are given any type of grain, these nutrients decrease tremendously and even disappear. Meat from grass-fed animals has two to four times more omega-3 essential fatty acids than meat from grain-fed animals.

These essential fats have slowed the growth of many malignant tumors and also kept them from spreading. Omega-3s can slow or even reverse the extreme weight loss that comes from advanced cancer. I believe if all meat-eaters switched from grain-fed to grass-fed meat, our national epidemic of obesity just might diminish. Seventy percent of the essential fatty acids in grass are omega-3s.

Unfortunately, when cattle are taken off omega-3-rich grass and shipped to a factory farm to be fattened up on grain, they begin losing their store of this beneficial fat. Each day that an animal spends in the feedlot, its supply of omega-3s diminishes. The ratio of omega-3 to omega-6 becomes extremely unbalanced, making grain-fed beef an inflammatory food.

Meat and dairy products from grass-fed cattle are the richest known source of another type of good fat, called *conjugated linoleic acid* or CLA. It consists of at least twenty-eight isomers. CLA is also known for its benefits to heart health since it has the ability to reduce inflammation and keep blood from becoming too thick.

Cows raised on fresh, green, plush, pasture alone have three to five times more CLA than products from animals fed a diet of just grain. CLA may be one of our most potent defenses against cancer and heart disease. Switching from grain-fed to grass-fed meat and dairy products may place you at a much lower cancer risk.

You can start by incorporating the following grass-fed products each day into your diet:

- One glass of certified, raw, grass-fed whole milk
- One ounce of raw cheese
- One serving of grass-fed meat

To approximate the same benefits from grain-fed meat and dairy products, you would have to eat five times that amount of grain, but you still wouldn't benefit as much.

In addition to being higher in omega-3s and CLA, meat and dairy from grass-fed animals is also higher in vitamin E. Vitamin E is another important heart-healthy nutrient. The meat from pastured cattle is four times higher in vitamin E than meat from the factory cattle. When humans consume grass-fed meats and dairy, the vitamin E content has been known to reduce their risk of heart disease and cancer.

Iron, zinc, calcium, and magnesium are all necessary minerals needed for healthy blood, bones, and teeth. These necessary minerals are present in grass-fed meats and dairy. Unfortunately, factory beef and dairy lose all these minerals almost immediately after being fed grain.

Creatine is a compound formed in protein that is necessary for building muscles. It is a nitrogenous organic compound that occurs naturally in vertebrates and helps supply energy to all cells in the body, mostly muscle. Creatine found in grass-fed meats and dairy partitions toward muscle mass in the human body when consumed. With the consumption of grain-fed meats, the creatine is diminished, and therefore the meat partitions in our bodies toward storing fat rather than muscle mass.

Oh Deer! Another Healthy Meat

Venison comes from animals, such as our native white-tailed deer, reindeer, moose, elk, and several nonnative animals such as red deer, axis deer, fallow deer, sika deer, blackbuck antelope, and nilgai antelope.

What Are the Health Benefits of Venison?

There are no additives or hormones in venison, unlike most factory farming in which animals are raised under intense pressure to pack on the pounds as quickly as possible while being pumped with growth hormones. Wild deer live a free and natural life without any hormones, additives, or antibiotics, the way nature intended. They live and grow healthfully in a wild environment with a diet consisting of berries, wild grasses, and other forage. This diet creates meat that is abundant in the heart-healthy omega-3s.

As with other pastured animals, venison is also high in CLA. Venison is bounteous in vitamin E, calcium, and magnesium — all necessary for strong bones, a healthy heart, and for boosting memory and concentration. Venison is also rich in iron, a critical mineral for oxygen in the blood, and zinc for healthy immune function.

Bone Broths

Bone broth is an ancient healing food that has been used or thousands of years to heal the sick, as well as maintain optimal health. Bone broth is rich in healing nutrients, such as collagen, proline, glutamine, glycine, minerals, gelatin and enzymes, all known to support the immune system. These vital nutrients, abundant in bone broth, heal your gut lining and reduce intestinal inflammation. This may be why bone broth is highly recommended for digestive disorders.

Bone broth also supports skin, hair, muscles, tissues, joints, and bone mineral density. Bone broths are typically made from the bones and carcass of pasture-fed beef, deer, and chickens and may contain a small amount of meat adhering to the bones. The nutrients in bone broths are easily absorbed, which makes them extremely beneficial for those suffering from chronic conditions, such as Crohn`s disease and cancer. I believe bone broths are one of the most nutrient-dense superfoods on the planet.

A Final Thought

I thank you for reading this chapter; I know how sad and painful it has been to learn the horror of the factory-farming industry. Animals were certainly not meant to suffer, especially not for food and profit. I do believe that they are brought here as a gift by our loving God to bring us love and for us to return love unto them. Animals want to give and receive love no differently than any human.

CHAPTER SEVEN

Real, Raw, Humanely Raised Dairy: Nature's Most Perfect Food

The information in this chapter addresses many of the common questions my patients have asked on a regular basis.

What Is Raw Milk?

Raw milk is unpasteurized and nonhomogenized.

Raw milk comes from healthy cows that are grazing on pasture and contains all the biodiversity of beneficial bacteria, fats, proteins, vitamins, and minerals. Raw milk has not been processed or altered from its original state in any way.

Raw milk from a clean, grass-fed cow was once known as nature's most perfect food. The inhumane, unsanitary conditions, and rapid production of milk led to the rise in sickness in humans who drank the product.

Raw milk contains many live active components that naturally have the ability to kill pathogenic bacteria and strengthen the immune system. These many components are packed with all the vital and critical benefits that make raw dairy a perfect food.

Here is the beneficial list of healthy proteins, good bacteria, and digestible proteins present before pasteurization destruction:

- Lacto-peroxidase
- Lacto-ferrin
- Antimicrobial components of blood (leukocytes, B-macrophages, neutrophils, T-lymphocytes, immunoglobulins and antibodies)
- Special carbohydrates (polysaccharides and oligosaccharides)
- Special fats (medium-chain fatty acids, phospholipids, and spingolipids)
- Complement enzymes
- Lysozyme
- Hormones
- Growth factors
- Mucins
- Fibronectin
- Glycomacropeptide
- Beneficial bacteria
- Bifidus factor
- B12-binding protein

What Is Pasteurization?

Pasteurization is a process that was developed in the late 1800s by Louis Pasteur, a French chemist and microbiologist renowned for his discoveries of the principles of microbial fermentation and pasteurization.

Pasteurization heats the milk at a high temperature to destroy any unfriendly microbes that have the potential for causing sickness. The obvious reason for using Pasteur's high-heat procedure was to allow milk farmers to catch up with the massive milk production industry. Farmers had plenty of milk quantity, but not good quality. Heating the milk to any temperature above 140°F has the potential to destroy friendly bacteria and valuable nutrients, making this an unhealthy product.

The damaging heat of pasteurization and ultra-pasteurization largely inactivates raw milk's life-giving components. It destroys the many beneficial bioactive components necessary for a healthy digestion. Pasteurization turns the sugar of milk, known as *lactose*, into *beta-lactose*, which is far more soluble and therefore more rapidly absorbed in the system, increasing hunger. This creates a condition called *lactose intolerance*, which I believe is actually *pasteurization* intolerance.

Pasteurized dairy is a highly intolerable food due to the depletion of naturally occurring digestive enzymes that are destroyed through high heat. The physiology of raw milk is destroyed through pasteurization, making this food difficult to digest.

Got Milk?

Pasteurization is not the answer to fix the problem, simply because it leads to other health concerns. We've been drinking this poison for years thinking it was a safer, healthier choice over raw milk. When cows are treated humanely in a healthy and happy farm setting, raw milk can be an extremely beneficial food.

Pasteurization is one of the worst offenses of milk production, due to the destruction of all the vital nutrients. Pasteurization also destroys 40 percent of the iodine present in raw milk, making milk extremely intolerable.

Some of the problems caused by pasteurization are:

- Constipation
- Diarrhea
- Bone loss
- Digestive issues, such as colitis, Crohn's disease, and irritable bowel syndrome

High-Temperature Pasteurization

Milk is heated to 161°F for thirty-one seconds to sterilize the milk and kill bad bacteria. The problem with this process is that it also destroys all the healthy microorganisms or good bacteria. It destroys the enzymes necessary for digestion, as well as denatures the milk protein, making the product completely unavailable for proper digestive assimilation.

Consumption of high-heat pasteurized products leads to inflammatory conditions, including:

- Acid reflux
- Gas
- Bloating
- Inflammatory bowel disease
- Allergies
- Asthma

I highly recommend that you avoid products that are high-heat pasteurized.

Ultra-Pasteurized

Ultra-pasteurization heats the milk to 280°F–300°F for only a few seconds and then chills it rapidly. The reason for using ultra-pasteurization is because it destroys everything. This process kills potentially harmful bacteria in the milk, and also damages all the vitamins, minerals, and other vital nutrients originally found in the milk. Ultra-pasteurized products are typically found in most supermarkets since this process extends shelf life for profit. Lactose intolerance is a common issue for drinkers of ultra-pasteurized milk.

The absence of enzymes makes it virtually impossible to ferment the milk for cultured products like yogurt and kefir. Enzymes are necessary for the culturing process; however, these live active components have died off in the ultra-heat process. During the ultra-pasteurization process, a test is performed to destroy phosphatase, a beneficial compound found in dairy. I highly suggest that you completely avoid ultra-pasteurized milk and this includes organic ultra-pasteurized as well.

Low-Temp Pasteurization

Unlike ultra- and high-heat processing, milk is only heated to 145°F and is cooled as quickly as possible. This temperature allows most of the nutrients and enzymes to stay intact. This processing is called *vat pasteurization*. In vat pasteurization, the milk is usually not homogenized, which means the cream line at the top of the milk is still as nature intended. This temperature doesn't have the potential to cause protein destruction, as does ultra- and high-heat pasteurization. The problem with low-temp pasteurization is that some of the necessary enzymes and probiotics may still suffer some assault.

Certified raw milk from a humanely raised source is always best because the milk is exactly the way the Creator intended. As you continue this chapter, you will learn the myths and truth about dairy.

Casein- or Lactose-Intolerance

As mentioned previously, pasteurization destroys *L. lactis* and other lactic-acid bacteria in milk. Let's take a closer look at what that means. These beneficial bacteria produce enzymes that break down the *casein* molecule. Milk allergy or milk intolerance is caused by casein intolerance, almost always from pasteurized dairy. There are reportedly testimonials of some autistic children being able to completely reverse their symptoms with the benefits of raw milk.

Lactose is the primary carbohydrate found in cow's milk. Lactose is made from one molecule of two simple sugars: glucose and galactose. People with lactose intolerance do not make the enzyme lactase and cannot digest milk sugar. Raw milk has its lactose-digesting Lactobacilli bacteria intact since it has not been destroyed through pasteurization. This may allow people who have avoided milk to consume and enjoy raw milk without ill effects.

Homogenization

Homogenization is the process that destroys the beautifully separated butterfat by breaking up the fat molecules into smaller droplets that remain suspended in the milk rather than rising to the top. This is achieved by driving the milk and cream through tiny holes using high heat and pressure. The process changes the molecular structure of the milk and possibly changes the way we are able to digest the milk.

Homogenizing leaves the milk virtually absent of the cream line at the top due to the breakdown of molecules. This damaging process then forms a compound called *xanthine oxidase* or XO, a major contributor to heart disease. This is due to the oxidation of the fat and cholesterol in the cream line.

Does Raw Milk Go Bad?

If you leave typical pasteurized milk unrefrigerated for a period of time, it can putrefy and create botulism, a *clostridium botulinum bacterium*, making one sick if consumed. If you leave raw milk unrefrigerated, it will turn into a nutrient-dense, cultured food. You can separate the cream and make butter, buttermilk, yogurt, and whey. You can add kefir grains to make a probiotic-rich beverage. Raw milk contains all the live active components keeping the milk from rotting, whereas dead milk can no longer survive from the deactivation of beneficial bacteria and enzymes through pasteurization.

A Note on Natural Hormones

Hormones are healthy, normal constituents of milk, called *peptides*, produced in one tissue, transported by blood, to cause another target tissue or organ to modify growth, metabolism, or reproduction. Hormones are essential for growth in humans and animals and can be transferred in small amounts from the blood into milk.

Raw milk contains these naturally occurring active hormones, including growth hormones. Please be aware that these bioactive forms of naturally occurring growth hormones present in both raw and pasteurized dairy products have no harmful effects when consumed by humans. Naturally occurring hormones found in cow milk have been sold as a hormone supplement to successfully treat those suffering from growth issues.

In summary, growth hormones in cow's milk are only harmful to humans when a lactating cow is injected with artificial growth hormones such as RGBh, recombinant bovine growth hormone, a poisonous growth hormone that has been linked to early menstruation and estrogen-dominant type cancers. To ensure that you are purchasing milk that does not contain RGBh, please consider certified raw milk farms. Search for a farm near you at www.realmilk.com.

A Perfect Food the Way the Creator Intended

These components have many benefits, such as destroying pathogens in the milk while stimulating the immune system. *Lactoferrin* is responsible for a healthy gut wall, prevents absorption of pathogens and toxins in the gut, and ensures assimilation of all the vital nutrients found in raw milk. The anti-microbial effect of raw milk is so powerful that even when large quantities of pathogenic bacteria are present in raw milk, they completely diminish over time.

The Negative Phosphatase

The mammary cells present in raw cow's milk produce an enzyme called *phosphatase*. Phosphatase is a naturally occurring beneficial enzyme that is important for healthy bones. The consumption of these ultra-pasteurized dairy products has been linked to the depletion of bone mineral density. The phosphatase enzyme is also important for the digestion of lactose, a naturally occurring milk sugar.

Immediately after pasteurization, the farmer conducts a phosphatase test to confirm that pasteurization has succeeded. Because phosphatase is naturally occurring in raw milk, the negative phosphatase test will detect the difference between raw milk and pasteurized milk.

A milk phosphatase kit is used for detecting the presence of enzymes. The test is based on yellow color, which is developed when phosphatase is active in the milk. The phosphatase enzyme is inactivated when pasteurization is carried out at 72°C or 161.6°F for fifteen seconds. This test takes about five minutes to determine if the enzyme is present in milk. If phosphatase is still present, then more heat will be applied until this beneficial compound is totally destroyed.

Processing for Profit

Not only does pasteurization and homogenization destroy all the bioactive benefits and valuable nutrients in dairy, but it also extends shelf life for profit. Back in the late 1800s, we were becoming an industrialized civilization. Farmers were mass-producing milk to keep up with the industry. This massive production of dairy and inhumane farming practices created infectious-filled milk.

Consumption of raw milk caused many people to get sick, which influenced the need for pasteurization. Cattle were often fed waste grain products from distilleries, leading to illness in the cattle and in humans who drank their milk. Louis Pasteur, a French chemist and microbiologist, discovered the principles of microbial fermentation and pasteurization. A law requiring pasteurization was passed around 1864. Pasteurization is used today to destroy pathogens found in dairy products. These pathogens are a direct result of inhumane, unsanitary farming practices. Pasteurization is obviously not a method used for safety, but for mass production and profit.

Nature's Most Perfect Food

Is dairy necessary in the human diet? That is a controversial question. The truth is that commercial, pasteurized milk and milk products have been associated with health problems. Raw dairy, however, is altogether different in its effects on the body and is a highly valuable food. Raw, pasture-raised dairy is such a complete food that one can live off of it exclusively, as it has the ability to satisfy every nutritional need.

Cow Milk: Only for Baby Calves?

Let me make something clear: raw dairy is not only for baby calves as some claim. Raw dairy was an important food in biblical and ancient times. Patriarchs like Isaac, Abraham, and Jacob lived off their herds of cattle and were noted as the healthiest people on the planet. Even Jesus drank milk; therefore, it's good enough for me.

As I discovered the answer to my personal healing, raw dairy was one of the foods that had a huge impact on my body's healing. The life-giving compounds restored my bone mineral density, as well as the live active components mentioned above, restoring my gut health.

Happy, healthy cows that graze on pasture are free of hormones, antibiotics, artificial insemination, and genetically modified feed, allowing their milk to be close to the milk consumed in ancient times. Factory-farmed milk production is not for anyone, as this is cruel, evil, and unfair to the precious animal, as well as the consumer. You have already learned the detrimental effects of pasteurized, inhumanely treated dairy in the above paragraphs. Let us not confuse one for the other.

...honey, curds, sheep, and cheese of the herd, for David and for the people who were with him, to eat; for they said, "The people are hungry and weary and thirsty in the wilderness."

—2 Samuel 17:29 NAS

The Land of Milk and Honey

In ancient and biblical times, refrigeration was not available. Milk was consumed fresh, made into butter, or cultured into products similar to cheese, cottage cheese, kefir, and yogurt. Milk is mentioned in the Bible in several places as an extremely beneficial and cultured food for human consumption.

Abraham gave milk to visiting angels.

And he took butter, and milk, and the calf which he had dressed, and set it before them; and he stood by them under the tree and they did eat.

—Genesis 18:8 KJV

Milk is used as a symbol of abundance, enjoyment, and nourishment.

Come, all you who are thirsty, come to the waters; and you who have no money, come, buy and eat! Come buy wine and milk without money and without cost.

—Isaiah 55:1 NIV

God used it to describe that land into which the Israelites would be brought.

*So I have come down to rescue them from the hand of the
Egyptians and to bring them up out of that land into a good
and spacious land, a land flowing with milk and honey.*
                                    —Exodus 3:8 NIV

Please keep in mind that these verses are referring to milk in
its God-given natural, raw, unadulterated state. Butter is also
high in vital nutrients. We will look at the abundance of health-
promoting nutrients in butter in the section on fats and oils.

God gave us milk in a superior, whole, health-promoting
form that is easily recognized and metabolized by our bodies.
We should consume milk as close to that form as possible.
Whenever humans interfere and alter what God has made,
we cause destruction and call it progress. The practice of
pasteurizing and homogenizing milk from cattle fed and raised
in confinement goes totally against what God intended.

It is not always easy to find raw milk and if you cannot find any
near you, it would be better that you consume no milk at all
than to consume commercial milk or even organic, pasteurized
milk. When looking for real, raw dairy products, please only
purchase from farms that are certified by the state to assure you
that the farmer is using humane and sanitary farming methods.

What About Organic Milk?

Organic milk does not mean raw. Milk that is labeled as only
organic is not a healthy choice. Organic milk products only mean
that the cows are given organic feed, so don't be deceived by
the marketing. These cows may still live in confinement, unable
to graze on pasture and enjoy the salad bar of nature.

Here are some of the life-giving aspects of raw, grass-fed dairy:

Healthy Bones and Teeth: Real milk and dairy products provide calcium, phosphorous, magnesium, and protein, all of which are critical for growth and development of healthy bone mineral density. Real, raw, grass-fed dairy taken from as early as childhood may contribute to strong bones and protect against diseases like osteoporosis later in life.

Keep in mind that vegetables in general contain large amounts of calcium; therefore, raw milk from pasture-raised cows is liquid calcium, so to speak. This form of plant-based calcium is extremely beneficial for the development and maintenance of healthy teeth and bones.

The amounts of calcium and phosphorous in raw dairy have been shown to help remineralize teeth from the effects of tooth decay.

When the teeth are exposed to acids in the mouth, the most abundant protein in milk is casein, and it is protective. It forms a thin film on the enamel surface. Casein prevents loss of calcium and phosphate from the enamel.

Did you know that the Royal Family of Great Britain has reportedly consumed fresh raw milk more than six hundred years? Also, indigenous peoples have consumed fresh whole milk for at least ten thousand years and most importantly, Jesus Christ advocated consuming milk from pasture-fed animals (Paige, 2013). This is a highly valuable, ancient, nutrient-rich food source when consumed in its natural, nonpasteurized, nonhomogenized form.

Obesity: The consumption of raw, whole dairy foods as part of a waist-watching diet is associated with increased weight loss.

There are naturally occurring enzymes found in milk fat that benefit the digestion process. Excess fat around the mid-section of the body is associated with greater risks to health. Therefore, people who consume raw, whole-dairy foods are more likely to be slimmer than those who consume low-fat foods.

Type 2 Diabetes: The consumption of raw dairy products may reduce the risk of type 2 diabetes, which has been a growing problem in the last fifty years.

Raw dairy foods have a low glycemic index, which helps to control blood glucose levels. This may be due to the effects of beneficial nutrients for a healthy pancreas.

Raw Dairy, Heart Disease, and Cancer: Fat-soluble vitamins A, D, and K2 in raw milk only come from cows grazing on pasture. Research has shown that raw dairy contains a higher level of these heart-healthy, anticancer compounds and fat-soluble vitamins.

Calcium and the naturally occurring fat in raw dairy products, known as Conjugated Linoleic Acid (CLA), have been noted for their protective components in breast, colon, bladder, prostate, and stomach cancers. CLA is also known for its anti-inflammatory agents and the reduction of cardiovascular disease.

Raw Milk — The Ultimate Thirst Quencher

For proper hydration, it is recommended that we consume approximately six to eight cups of water each day. Dehydration can result in poor memory and concentration, irritability, headaches, stomach issues, skin problem, and excessive hunger. Raw dairy contains many hydrating factors, such as enzymes and immunoglobulins, that replace electrolytes and satisfy thirst.

> *He said to her, "Please give me a little water to drink, for I am thirsty." So she opened a bottle of milk and gave him a drink; then she covered him.*
> —Judges 4:19 NAS

Let the Raw Truth Be Told

Due to the controversy surrounding raw dairy, safety may still be a concern for you. Let me explain and ease your fear from the negative ideas that the Food and Drug Administration (FDA) may have conditioned you to believe.

The growth and development of children who were fed raw milk were superior to those who consumed pasteurized, homogenized milk and milk products. Children fed raw milk were proven to have greater resistance to tuberculosis, scurvy, flu, diphtheria, pneumonia, asthma, allergies, skin problems, tooth decay, and bone and development issues.

What Is Cultured or Fermented Dairy?

Fermented or cultured dairy products are dairy foods that have fermented and developed lactic acid bacteria, such as *Lactobacillus, Lactococcus*, and *Leuconostoc*, making the milk a more digestible food.

Most common dairy companies synthetically add cultures back to the food after pasteurization. I like to call this process *dairy on CPR* or trying to bring food back to life after it has been destroyed.

You're probably disappointed at this point since you may have been consuming commercial dairy products, but *it's never too late* to make simple dietary changes that will bring forth great health benefits.

Many of these so-called cultured products found in grocery stores are nothing but impostors of probiotic-rich foods. Some of most the unhealthful, highly processed foods are conventional dairy. These include regular, fat-free, and reduced-fat yogurts, cheeses, milk products, ice-cream, half-and-half, and heavy cream. These products are laden with artificial growth hormones, synthetic vitamins, and are extremely indigestible.

Let's take a good look at the some of the raw, cultured dairy products that have been consumed for centuries. These are also some of the life-giving, probiotic rich foods that have restored my health.

Kefir and Yogurt from Raw Dairy

Kefir means *feel good* in Turkish. Kefir is an ancient food that is made by culturing milk. Culturing milk is simple; as a matter of fact, this process is done every twenty-four hours at my home. I love kefir for its creamy texture and life-giving beneficial probiotics that I believe contributed to my healing. Kefir is similar to yogurt, but a more liquid beverage. Drinking kefir is a wonderful way to ultimately restore your gut flora, even in the most critical gut environment. Raw kefir grains are the original and superior way of culturing dairy.

Here is how it's done:

> Place approximately 16 ounces of raw milk in a clean mason jar with two tablespoons of live kefir grains, then

cover the mason jar with a paper towel for 24 hours in your cupboard.

After culturing is complete, remove the kefir grains by straining them from what is now a cultured product.

This cultured product can now be enjoyed as a high-probiotic beverage.

Store kefir in refrigerator for up to two weeks in a glass mason jar. The remaining grains can be reused over and over by repeating the process. The grains will multiply every ten days and the extras may be eaten for a probiotic boost.

Reserve two tablespoons of grains for each batch of cultured milk.

The milk can be from cows, goats, sheep, or even coconuts. Kefir has a refreshing, slightly sour taste and is easily digested. Even those with dairy sensitivities can drink kefir due to the abundance of friendly probiotic strains that are used in the culturing process. These friendly organisms consume the lactose in the milk, making it a predigested food. Kefir grains are live bacteria or curds that are the necessary component for culturing. Kefir grains can be found at www.kefirlady.com.

Kefir contains many beneficial probiotic bacteria, as well as yeast, vitamins, minerals, and complete proteins. I like to call kefir *the giver of life* since raw kefir contains approximately sixty probiotics in each eight ounce cup, whereas yogurt contains seven to fifteen probiotics per eight ounces.

Kefir grains look similar in appearance to cauliflower. These grains are live active cultures that contain all necessary and beneficial bacteria, including lactic acid, which is needed for healthy fermentation.

Commercial kits that use powdered kefir are usually gleaned from pasteurized dairy and do not contain the necessary enzymes and bacteria for proper culturing.

Whey Protein from Raw Dairy

Whey is a by-product of cheese-making that was used as a therapeutic beverage for human nutrition in ancient Greece. Hippocrates prescribed fresh whey for many ailments. During the Middle Ages, many doctors successfully used whey for a variety of diseases. Whey was used throughout Central Europe to treat dyspepsia, uremia, arthritis, gout, liver disease, anemia, and tuberculosis. Today, whey is commonly used in cheese-making and whey protein shakes. Whey, as with all dairy products, should come from healthy, humanely raised cattle and be consumed raw.

The Bible says in Isaiah 7:15 that Jesus (Immanuel) would eat curds and honey so he would know to refuse evil and choose well. If Jesus Christ, who is fully God and fully man, needs to eat curds and honey, I need it more!

Raw Cheese

Raw cheeses are produced from raw milk, contain all the necessary enzymes, and are easily digested compared with those made from pasteurized milk. They also contain more bioavailable components just as raw milk does.

Not all cheeses labeled as "raw" are truly so. Though making cheese does require some heating, it can be done at very low temperatures that will preserve the nutritional integrity of the product. The body temperature of a cow is 101.5°F; therefore, milk heated to that temperature is still considered raw. Some companies heat the milk for their cheese products to just below the pasteurization temperature, which is extremely destructive to the compounds in milk. They are then allowed, legally, to present the cheese as "raw" because the milk was never brought all the way up to the pasteurization temperature. But this is not actually raw. When looking for real, raw cheese, the words *raw milk cheese*, not just *raw*, will assure you that your cheese contains all the necessary and valuable nutrients that qualify.

Also, keep in mind that emulsifiers, extenders, phosphates, and hydrogenated oils are added to processed cheeses. These should be completely avoided at all cost.

> *Bring also these ten cuts of cheese to the commander of their thousand, and look into the welfare of your brothers, and bring back news of them.*
> —1 Samuel 17:18 NAS

Butter Is Better

Butter and ghee are two of my favorite foods. I was so excited when I discovered the healing benefits of real butter. To think all the time I wasted, avoiding this delicious, highly nutritious superfood, believing that it was going to make me fat and clog my arteries.

Yes, butter is an excellent source of vitamins.

Butter is loaded with a wide range of health-giving properties. Butter contains an abundance of fat-soluble vitamins, such as vitamins A, D, E and K. Trace minerals, such as manganese, chromium, zinc, copper, and selenium, are found in butter, which is an extremely potent source of antioxidants. Butter is also a great source of iodine, making it beneficial for the thyroid.

Butter contains immune-supporting nutrients, as well as boosting the metabolism. It even has antimicrobial properties and is a delicious way to combat pathogenic microorganisms that live inside the intestinal tract.

> *He asked water, and she gave him milk; she brought forth butter in a lordly dish.*
>
> —Judges 5:25 KJV

Glycospingolipids

A type of beneficial fatty acids that specifically function to protect the stomach from gastrointestinal infections, *glycospingolipids* are an excellent source of cholesterol. Basically, cholesterol is a repair substance needed for healthy cellular activity. Cholesterol also plays a critical part in brain and nervous system development.

Butter is another wonderful heat-stable cooking staple due to its saturated fatty acids. Yes, you read that right.

Butter, the Perfect Omega-3 to Omega-6 Ratio

Butter has the perfect balance of omega-3 and omega-6 fats. Butter contains Conjugated Linoleic Acid (CLA). If your butter source is from cows that graze on grass and natural forage, then it contains high levels of CLA. This compound can help protect against different types of cancer. CLA also helps the body retain muscle instead of fat.

Butter is loaded with trace minerals, such as manganese, chromium, zinc, iodine, copper, and selenium, which are powerful antioxidants. You can get your required dose of short- and medium-chain fatty acids from butter, which are great for supporting your immune system and boosting metabolism. It also has antimicrobial properties, which are excellent for combating pathogenic bacteria that reside in your colon and intestines.

The Brain Is Made Up of Fat and Cholesterol

Butter is an excellent source of cholesterol. Your body needs dietary cholesterol for healthy cellular function. It also plays a critical part in the development of the brain and nervous system. So yes! Please eat butter for a healthy brain. The saturated fat in butter is a precursor to serotonin, oxytocin, endorphins, and dopamine, critical hormones that are responsible for your happiness. I believe that knowing butter is good for you is making you quite happy right about now.

Last but not least, butter, which comes from cows and not a chemist, contains the *Wulzen Factor*. This is a hormone-like substance with many functions. It can prevent stiffness in the joints, as well as arthritis. It is also responsible for ensuring that calcium is deposited in the bones rather than in the joints. Please be aware that the Wulzen Factor can only be found in raw butter and raw cream. Pasteurization totally destroys the Wulzen Factor. The Wulzen Factor, or anti-stiffness factor, was founded by Dutch researcher, Rosalind Wulzen, who discovered its benefits against calcification of the joints, as well as hardening of the arteries, cataracts, and calcification of the pineal gland. Butter should be from grass-fed cows and be organic, or raw and grass-fed, which is best. Sources for butter can be found in the resource section of this book.

Ghee or Clarified Butter

The definition of ghee, as stated by Omics International:

> Ghee is a class of clarified butter that originated in ancient India and is commonly used in Kurdish, Afghani, Pakistani, Indian, Bangladeshi, Nepali and Sri Lankan cuisine, traditional medicine, and religious rituals. (Omics International, 2014)

The impurities and dairy solids have been removed, so people who are lactose intolerant usually have virtually no problems consuming ghee. Ghee doesn't need to be refrigerated, and some mixtures can last even as long as a century.

Ghee, like butter, is also rich in healthy fat-soluble vitamins such as vitamins A, E, D, and K. I use ghee as part of my healthy fat intake on vegetables, sprouted whole-grain breads, and cooking. Ghee has a high smoking point, which makes it a good source for cooking and baking. Ghee cooks at a higher point than almost any other oil, and will not create free radical damage. Free radicals can potentially be harmful to one's health, and when oil smokes, it can be hazardous to a person's respiratory system if consistently breathed in.

Ghee is beneficial to intestinal bacteria, so those who suffer from digestive disorders will benefit greatly. It also helps to increase appetite, and when ghee is from healthy grass-fed cows, the butter contains the cancer-fighting fatty acid CLA.

> *For the churning of milk produces butter, and pressing the nose brings forth blood; so the churning of anger produces strife.*
>
> —Proverbs 30:33 NAS

Bottom Line

As far as finding real dairy that is similar to the quality explained in this segment, I suggest that you always speak to the farmer about what the cows are eating, how much sunlight they receive each day, and most importantly, if the farmer is certified by the state. The only way to assure safety is to search for certified raw, grass-fed dairy.

Dr. Weston Andrew Valleau Price was a dentist in the late 1800s. He was primarily known for his theories on the relationships between nutrition, dental health, and physical health. Living in Cleveland, Price was called the *Isaac Newton of Nutrition*. For additional reading, I suggest his book, *Nutrition and Physical Denegation*, originally published in 1939.

I also highly suggest The Weston Price Foundation at www. realmilk.com. Weston A. Price was a true pioneer in holistic medicine, and I learned much of my nutritional information from his work. I highly recommend that you research Dr. Price.

CHAPTER EIGHT

Nondairy Milks

Soy Is NOT a health food!

I believe one of the biggest dietary mistakes is the consumption of soy products, including soy milk. Many people have removed cow milk and replaced it with soy milk, mostly due to their intolerance of processed milk.

Ever wonder why there is such a rise in early puberty with young girls starting their menstrual cycle at ages as young as six and seven? Even little boys have shown enlarged breasts and early development. According to the American Academy of Pediatrics, 25 percent of infants are on soy formula, which could jeopardize brain and body development, and are at high risk for different types of cancers. I have worked successfully with many young patients who suffered from the effects of soy infant formula.

Studies have shown that infants who consume soy formula are consuming an abundance of excess hormones equivalent to four birth control pills a day.

We were led to believe that soy was a large part of Asian cuisine; however, it was only used as a condiment in the form of *fermented* soy, which includes tempeh, miso, and natto, used only in small quantities. Fermenting the soy removed the phytic acid that is the naturally accruing anti-nutrient present in soybeans. These anti-nutrients cause a host of health issues. Soy contains calcium, magnesium, copper, iron, and zinc.

High levels of phytic acid in soy reduce the ability to assimilate these minerals, which is why gas and bloating occur when soy is consumed. These important minerals become trapped in the intestines, resulting in mineral deficiencies. Diets high in phytic acid have caused growth problems in children. Soy foods also contain high levels of aluminum, which is toxic to the brain and nervous system, liver, and kidneys.

Keep in mind that the soybean did not serve as a food until the discovery of this fermentation process sometime during the Chou Dynasty. Tofu, known as *bean curd*, was also a product that was discovered around the second century BCE (before common era). The Chinese did not eat any unfermented soybeans, which contain large quantities of these natural toxins known as enzyme inhibitors or anti-nutrients. These enzyme inhibitors block the absorption of trypsin and other enzymes needed for protein digestion, making unfermented soy extremely difficult to digest.

These inhibitors can produce serious gastric distress, such as bloating, indigestion, and discomfort. Diets high in trypsin inhibitors cause enlargement and pathological conditions of the pancreas, including cancer. Unfermented soybeans contain *hemagglutinin*, a clot-promoting substance that causes blood cells to clot together, contributing to heart disease and stroke.

Scientific studies have identified that rats fed soy fail to grow normally. The Chinese began to incorporate the soybean after the discovery of how to ferment it. Soy's depressant compound, such as phytic acid, is greatly deactivated during the process of fermentation.

Historically, the Chinese never consumed modern soy milk, soy butter, soy cheese, or soy-isolated protein.

Soy contains higher levels of *phytoestrogens* than any other food source. Phytoestrogens are plant-based estrogens that mimic estrogen in our bodies. You may have read studies that indicate phytoestrogens are good for you. The soy industry funded these studies in order to sell more soy. Independent research clearly indicates that unfermented soy consumption is extremely unhealthy.

One of the leading causes of breast cancer, thyroid conditions, endometriosis, uterine fibroids, infertility, and low libido is *unopposed estrogen*, or *estrogen dominance*, which is present in patients with these conditions. Yes, I know, you're shaking your head in disbelief, but it doesn't end there.

My dear friends, you may know someone, or perhaps even you have thyroid issues, such as hypo- or hyperthyroidism, weight gain, digestive problems, or some form of cancer, all of which have a direct link to soy consumption. You may also experience mood swings, dry skin, chronic fatigue syndrome, digestive upset, and you may be one of those people who feel cold most of the time.

Soy has a detrimental effect on your thyroid, due to the thyroid-suppressing *goitrogens*. Goitrogens are substances that interfere with iodine uptake in the thyroid gland. Soy actually prevents your thyroid from absorbing iodine, a necessary element for thyroid function.

Another issue with soy products is allergies that result from your immune system recognizing part of the food as a harmful, foreign substance and then attacking it. This is called a *xenoestrogen effect*. Xenoestrogens are products that mimic estrogen and are foreign to the body. Their presence results in disease. Allergies to soy products are extremely common. Usually symptoms of a soy allergy may be tingling in the mouth, itchy skin, swelling, abdominal pain, headache, runny nose, congestion, or even problems breathing.

In response to the allergen, your body releases into your bloodstream histamines and other chemicals, producing these allergy symptoms.

I find that most people usually say that they do not consume soy, yet soy ingredients are hidden in more than 85 percent of prepackaged and processed foods. Most factory-farmed livestock consume soy grain products. As stated in an earlier section, remember that it's not only true that you are what you eat, but also that you are what your food eats.

Many fast food chains, as well as your favorite family-owned restaurants, could be cooking in soybean oil, and you wouldn't even know it.

Another serious health concern with soy is that 94 percent of soy is genetically modified. GMO soybeans may be linked to infant mortality and inability to conceive. GMO soy also generates dangers such as infertility, gastrointestinal complications, organ damage, immune-system problems, accelerated aging, and serious hormonal health issues that lead to cancer. Soy is genetically modified to be herbicide-resistant which means the crop can be treated with glyphosate-containing products without the crop being damaged.

If you would like to consume soy products, please look for organic soy to avoid genetic mutations. Please be sure to consume soy only in the fermented form to ensure better digestion and assimilation. Remember that soy fermentation converts minerals such as calcium, iron, magnesium, potassium, selenium, copper, and zinc into more soluble forms and can also increase vitamin levels in the final product. Please consume organic, fermented soy products in small quantities. These include soy sauce, miso, natto, tempeh, and tamari.

Organic, fermented soy products can be found in the resource section at the back of this book.

Almond and Cashew Milk

Other popular nondairy milks are rice, hemp, almond, and cashew. Unlike soy milk, these nondairy products have beneficial value in their raw, unpasteurized form. Let's first examine nut milks, such as the popular almond and cashew. Organic is always best to avoid chemical fertilizers and genetic mutations; however, store-bought nut milks, even organic, are pasteurized. As with cow and goat dairy, nut milks are also best consumed raw to assure you of optimal nutrition as well as healthy digestion.

Now, you're probably wondering where to get raw nut milk. Making it yourself is your best option and not as difficult as you may think. Soaking the nuts makes the nutrients more bioavailable for better digestion and assimilation. Soaking successfully removes any enzyme inhibitors or phytic acid, present in most grains and nuts, making them easier to digest.

The bottom line is to stop buying store-bought nut milks, and this includes coconut and rice milk. I am not at all saying that nut milks are not good for you. I am saying that most store-bought milks are highly processed and contain added chemicals. They are pasteurized and contain many chemical-laden ingredients including artificial vitamins. Even the organic ones are still processed with unwanted ingredients and pasteurized to extend the shelf-life.

Most of the time, there is the equivalent of only a few nuts and mostly water in the store-bought versions. Additionally, *carrageenan*, a suspected cancer-causing ingredient, is added to most brands as a thickener. Carrageenan is not digested properly; and therefore, may be destructive to the digestive system. Consumption of carrageen overstimulates the immune system, which creates an inflammatory response and a possible link to colitis, intestinal lesions, and colon and gastrointestinal cancer.

Please enjoy my simple recipe for nut milk:

> Soak approximately 1 cup of raw organic almonds or cashews overnight, completely submerged in about 3-4 cups of warm water and ½ teaspoon of unrefined salt. The salt helps deactivate the phytic acid making the final result easier to assimilate.
>
> Leave the nut mixture uncovered on the counter for 8 hours or overnight.
>
> Drain nuts and spread on a baking sheet or dehydrator sheet and dry the nuts on the lowest temperature of 150°F. To successfully dehydrate the nuts, you will need twenty-four hours. This can be done in your conventional oven. If

you have a dehydrator you would use the same time and temperature.

Remove nuts from oven and allow to cool for an hour.

In a high-speed blender add:
1 cup of the nuts
2–3 cups of pure water or raw coconut water—I prefer
coconut water
A small amount of raw honey (optional)
1 teaspoon of pure, organic vanilla extract (optional)

Blend on high speed for 2–4 minutes, adding more liquid for a thinner consistency or less liquid for a thicker consistency.

Strain mixture into a large bowl through a cheese cloth or a dish towel.

The final product can be stored in a glass container for up to a week.

LET'S HEAD TO THE TROPICS

Coconut, the Fruit of Life

Coconuts and coconut milk are two of my personal favorites. Coconut is a fruit that provides a nutritious food, oil, and a drink. Coconuts are packed with various health benefits: nutrients, minerals, vitamins, and dietary fiber. Coconuts are also regarded as wonder foods because of their life-saving properties. They are also labeled as functional food because of their various health benefits.

Coconuts are a beneficial, staple food in many cultures all over the world. Coconut products have also been used as an effective traditional medicine for thousands of years. The health benefits of the coconut are numerous, and they give us a delicious creamy taste and texture. They are great for cooking, baking, and smoothies.

A Little Coconut History

Coconuts are used in a variety of cuisines. They are primarily a tropical product with main production in Asia — Indonesia, the Philippines, and India. The coconut is a versatile fruit with a diverse use in both domestic and commercial industries.

Here are the top ten growers of coconuts:

1. Philippines
2. Indonesia
3. Brazil
4. India
5. Mexico
6. Vietnam
7. Papua New Guinea
8. Sri Lanka
9. Thailand
10. Tanzania

What Is Coconut Milk?

Coconut milk is the liquid from the grated meat of a coconut. It should not be confused with coconut water. The color and rich creamy texture and taste of coconut milk can be attributed to the high oil content. Most of the fat is saturated fat. In particular, the saturated fat, lauric acid, and medium-chain triglycerides in coconuts are extremely nourishing to the thyroid gland.

Coconuts and coconut milk have unnecessarily received a bad rap due to high saturated fat content. Despite the bad rap, island populations around the world have healthfully used the fruit's meat juice, milk, and oil in everything from cooking, skin and hair care to disease prevention. Furthermore, the unique fatty acids in coconut milk may aid in weight loss, reduce heart disease, improve skin and hair, balance the thyroid hormone, and improve immune function.

Please refer to chapter nine, "The Big Fat Lie About Fat and Cholesterol," of this book for more information on the benefits of saturated fat.

Coconut milk is quite different than coconut water, and many have mistaken the water for the milk. Coconut water has received a great deal of attention for its many health benefits and is an important treatment for acute diarrhea as well as most parasitic conditions of the gut. This highly nutritious, clear liquid has the same electrolyte balance as human blood plasma, making it an extremely valuable hydrating tonic before and after long periods of intensive exercise. When I attend a sports event at my daughter's school, it upsets me to see sugar- and chemical-laden sports drinks disguising as a *healthy* drink for the children. Coconut water has been known to successfully prevent dehydration and electrolyte loss without the use of harmful chemicals, artificial colors or flavors, or high sugar content.

Coconuts are known for fiber, vitamins C, E, B1, B3, B5 and B6 and minerals including iron, selenium, sodium, calcium, magnesium, and phosphorous. Most important, the medium chain fatty acids, or MCFAs, are rapidly metabolized into energy in the liver. Unlike other saturated fats, MCFAs are used up more quickly by the body and are less likely to be stored as fat.

Saturated fat from coconut may contribute to the prevention of coronary heart disease.

The fat in coconuts is mostly in the form of medium-chain saturated fatty acids (MCFAs), in particular, one called lauric acid. Lauric acid is converted by the liver into a highly beneficial compound called *monolaurin*, a natural antiviral substance in coconut milk that retards the growth of unfriendly microbes in the digestive tract. I like to call coconut products the antiviral food source.

Monolaurin is an antiviral, antifungal, and antibacterial agent that destroys a wide variety of diseases, which, in turn, contribute unfriendly organisms in the digestive tract. Over time, these unfriendly microbes may travel as pathogenic compounds into the blood. We know now that the consumption of coconut milk and other coconut products may help protect the body from infections, candida, and viruses. Enjoy your coconut milk. Aren't you excited now?

Coconut Products and Weight Loss

We took the fat out of the American diet, and we got fatter and sicker.

We now know that not eating enough good fat can actually make you fat. People who include healthy fats such as coconut products in their diets actually eat less than those who don't get enough fat. Good fats like coconut products satiate the brain receptors that control appetite. The saturated fat in coconut oil and full-fat coconut milk help the body feel full while reducing the appetite. This is the exact reason low fat diets make you crave carbohydrates and sugar. The nutrient density in saturated fat keeps you fuller longer while reducing your chance of cheating.

The fat in coconut milk and other coconut products increases metabolism and therefore aids in weight loss. The medium-chain triglycerides in coconut milk and coconut oil are the elements that sustain you longer, making you less susceptible to cravings. Cravings are usually an indication of a deficiency caused by fad diets.

When consuming coconut products, please always look for raw and organic, as this will ensure optimal flavor and highest nutritional value.

Let's Dive Into a Cup of Hemp Milk

Hemp milk or hemp-seed milk is highly nutritious. Made from adding water to hemp seeds that are soaked and ground, it yields a nutty, rich, and creamy beverage. Hemp milk has become popular in the holistic health industry as a great way to receive plant-based protein.

Some of the many benefits of hemp milk are as follows:

B Vitamins. Hemp milk supplies a sufficient amount of B vitamins, which help convert the food you eat into energy. Just one eight ounce cup of hemp milk supplies the RDA (recommended daily allowance) of 2.4 micrograms of vitamin B-12. Vitamin B-12 helps your body produce red blood cells, increases energy, and prevents anemia and damage to your nerves.

Vitamin D. That eight ounce cup of real hemp milk also supplies 30 percent of 1000 international units (IU) of vitamin D. Vitamin D helps your body effectively absorb calcium into the skeletal structure. Additionally, vitamin D is a precursor to *serotonin*, the feel-good hormone in the brain. Prolonged vitamin D deficiency has been linked to many types of cancer.

Children under five years of age need 35 IU of vitamin D per day. Children ages five to ten need 2500 units per day, and adults need 4000–8000 units per day. Pregnant woman need between 5000–10,000 units of vitamin D per day. Please check with your doctor for an accurate dosage of vitamin D for your personal needs.

Other Benefits. Hemp milk also strengthens the immune system. It helps build a strong and healthy heart, increases mental capacity, is vital for healthy clear skin and hair, and is abundant in anticancer compounds.

A Little History on Hemp

Hemp is one of the earliest known domesticated plants. It has been cultivated by many civilizations for more than twelve thousand years, yet remains popular today. Hemp use dates as far back as the Neolithic period in China, with hemp fiber imprints found on Yang Shao culture pottery dating from the fifth century BCE. The Chinese later used hemp to make ropes, clothing, and paper.

The world-leading producer of hemp is China with smaller production in Europe, Chile, and North Korea. According to cannibismedical.com, "While more hemp is exported to the United States than to any other country in the world, the United States government does not distinguish between marijuana and the non-psychoactive cannabis used for industrial and commercial purposes."

The best sources of coconut, hemp, and other nondairy products are included in the resource section of this book.

CHAPTER NINE

The Big Fat Lie About Fat and Cholesterol

Wake up America! STOP believing the Cholesterol Myth! Let's first talk about what cholesterol is, and why you need it.

That's right, you do need cholesterol.

What is cholesterol, besides being your best friend?

Cholesterol is a molecular-weight alcohol manufactured by the liver, measured in high-density lipoproteins—any group of soluble proteins that transport fat or lipids throughout the bloodstream—or LP(a)s, low-density LP(a)s, and triglycerides, as explained below.

High-Density Lipoprotein or **HDL**. HDL helps prevent heart disease by removing excess LDL and arterial plaque from your arteries.

Low-Density Lipoprotein or **LDL.** LDL circulates in your blood giving your cells the integrity and protection they need.

Triglycerides. This dangerous fat is converted into glucose or sugar which makes your body store fat. Thus, high levels of triglycerides are linked to diabetes and heart disease.

Triglyceride levels rise in response to:

- Eating processed grains and sugars
- Physical inactivity
- Smoking cigarettes
- Excessive alcohol consumption
- Obesity or carrying extra weight

Lipoprotein. Lipoproteins are made up of an LDL, which is a protein found in your blood, manufactured by the liver. The liver does not make mistakes, and that is why cholesterol is considered an antioxidant, protecting the body against oxidative stress that leads to free radical damage and disease.

There Is NO Bad or Good Cholesterol: It's All Good

Cholesterol is a precursor to hormones and constitutes every cell membrane in your body. It is needed for a healthy brain, which is why patients taking a statin drug (cholesterol-lowering drug) eventually develop disorders of the brain and central nervous system resulting in Alzheimer's disease or extreme forgetfulness. Cholesterol also plays a critical role in bones and teeth.

When a cholesterol-lowering drug is prescribed by a doctor, a host of health problems can occur. Typically, serotonin—the feel-good hormone in the brain—diminishes over time. Then a doctor may prescribe an antidepressant which contributes to other health issues. Joints become atrophied, numbness and stiffness occur—the list goes on. Dietary cholesterol from sources like eggs, coconut products, grass-fed meats, nuts and seeds, and raw dairy do not cause elevated cholesterol in your blood serum, but your doctor may very well tell you to avoid these beneficial and important foods.

Cholesterol repairs tissue and cell damage caused by a poor diet. If your body senses you are under attack— from consuming too much sugar in the forms of refined sugar and refined grains— it will raise your cholesterol levels. Most prepackaged snacks, reduced-fat and diet foods, and boxed cereal all convert to sugar, resulting in a body in need of repair.

Cholesterol, then, is your best friend, not the villain that we have been conditioned to believe. The only fats that are unhealthy are the trans fats known as *hydrogenated oils*.

Hydrogenated oils are corn oil, soybean oil, and canola oil. These are found in so-called *healthy* diet foods, highly processed dairy substitutes, and prepackaged food-like products packaged as healthy food sources. These inflammatory foods are the root cause of oxidative stress and cellular damage that lead to heart disease and cancer.

Inflammation Is the Cause of Heart Disease

Inflammation is a natural occurrence resulting from damage within the body. It is caused by a highly processed and refined-carbohydrate diet. The inflammatory response creates internal ballooning in the tissues, which then causes narrowing or thinning of your arteries. When the arteries become narrow, this process restricts blood and oxygen to the heart and brain. The medical term is hardening of the arteries, or *arteriosclerosis*, and it is often followed by an episode such as a heart attack or a stroke.

There is little to no cholesterol found in the arteries of a heart attack or stroke patient. Restricted blood flow from inflammation inside the body results in plaque buildup that leads to arterial damage known as *calcification*. This plaque, along with the thickening of your blood and constricting of your blood vessels that normally occur during the inflammatory process, increases your risk of high blood pressure and heart attacks.

Cholesterol levels then rise to replace your damaged cells since cholesterol is a necessary repair substance.

The real inflammatory markers of heart disease are *homocysteine levels* and *cardio reactive proteins* (CRP) levels. These inflammatory markers indicate heart disease, certainly not cholesterol.

Blaming Cholesterol for Heart Disease Is Like Blaming Police for Crime

Here's an easier way for you to understand the cholesterol and statin story. Imagine you're in a high-crime area, and you see large numbers of police responding. When your body creates inflammation due to a highly processed or unhealthy diet, it becomes a high crime area. Now cholesterol, like the police, begins to increase due to the excess amount of inflammation, as does the need for more officers when crime increases.

Now, I want you to think of crime as inflammation, and the police force as cholesterol. However, doctors often take out a gun and start shooting the police as if they are the reason for the crime. Taking a statin, known as a cholesterol-lowering drug, is no different than shooting the police when they are there to reduce the crime. Cholesterol arrives like a police force to reduce the inflammation caused by your diet. Remember, cholesterol is an inflammatory first responder, and when your body is under attack, cholesterol elevates to repair the damage.

Who Said Cholesterol Was the Villain?

Dr. Joseph Mercola writes in his article, "The Cholesterol Myth That Could Be Harming Your Health:"

> In 2004, the U.S. government's National Cholesterol Education Program panel advised those at risk for heart disease to attempt to reduce their LDL cholesterol to very specific, low levels.
>
> In 2003, a 130 milligram LDL cholesterol level was considered healthy. Updated guidelines set dangerously low levels of less than 100 milligrams, or even less than 70 for patients labeled high risk.
>
> Keep in mind that these extremely low targets often require dangerous multiple dosages of cholesterol-lowering drugs.
>
> Fortunately, in 2006, a review in the *Annals of Internal Medicine* found that there is insufficient evidence that support the target numbers outlined by the panel. The authors of this review study were unable to find any research providing evidence that achieving a specific LDL target level was important in and of itself. (Mercola, 2010)

The writers of the review went on to discover that the studies attempting to provide this evidence suffered from major flaws. Several of the scientists who developed these crazy guidelines admitted that the scientific evidence supporting the less-than-seventy-milligrams recommendation was weak.

How These Excessively Low Cholesterol Guidelines Developed

Approximately 90 percent of the doctors on the panel that developed the new cholesterol guidelines had been receiving money from drug companies that manufacture statin cholesterol-lowering drugs. Yes, I said it.

> Too much money is invested in statins for those in white lab coats to say otherwise. Unfortunately, cardiologists are finding out that their patients with cholesterol levels that are too low are left without protection from cholesterol. These patients are actually at risk for a heart attack or stroke.

> Despite the finding that there is absolutely no evidence at all to show that lowering LDL cholesterol to 100 or below is good for you, the American Heart Association still recommends lowering your LDL cholesterol levels to less than 100. (Mercola, 2010)

The prescribed treatment to lower cholesterol levels under 100 almost always includes one or more cholesterol-lowering drugs. I have many patients who come to me for help complaining about the symptoms caused by their statins. These patients are usually on two cholesterol-lowering drugs.

Statin Drugs Are a Medical Time Bomb in Modern Medicine

Statin drugs inhibit the production of cholesterol. They also hinder your body's production of *Coenzyme* Q10 (CoQ10). This antioxidant promotes heart health and muscle function. Rarely do doctors inform patients that they should take a CoQ10 supplement while taking a cholesterol-lowering drug. They then suffer a depletion that leads to fatigue, muscle weakness, soreness, and eventually heart failure.

Rhabdomyolysis, severe muscle pain and weakness, is the most common side effect of statin drugs, which include muscle atrophy and muscle pain.

In addition, statin drugs have an accumulative effect on cellular activity, typically causing cellular atrophy. Atrophy symptoms include:

- Muscle injury
- Stiffness
- Weakness
- Numbness

These symptoms indicate wasting away of cells. This may be an indication that your bodily tissues are breaking down which could eventually lead to organ damage and failure. Clearly, this process is the degeneration of cells or cell death.

Statin drugs have also been linked to the following:

- Polyneuropathy in hands and feet (pain and numbness)
- Dizziness
- Cognitive impairment, includes memory loss
- Risk of high blood sugar, type 2 diabetes
- Increased risk of cancer
- Decreased immune function
- An increase in liver enzymes
- Diminished serotonin, dopamine, and oxytocin (Mercola, 2010)

Perhaps this is why patients on a statin drug over time are normally prescribed an antidepressant.

The Lipid Hypothesis

The belief that low-fat concoctions and cholesterol-free foods are healthy is radically wrong. The brainwashing information that saturated fats cause heart disease as well as cancer is *mis*information. To understand, we must examine the exact chemistry of fats.

Fats, or lipids, are organic substances that are not soluble in water. Fatty acids are chains of carbon atoms with hydrogen atoms filling available bonds. The most common fat in our bodies and our food is triglycerides. A *triglyceride* is composed of three fatty-acid chains attached to a glycerol molecule.

A glycerol molecule is a carbohydrate that is made in the body through consumption of glucose. It exists in triglycerides. Elevated triglycerides in the blood have been positively linked to heart disease, but keep in mind, these triglycerides do not come from dietary fats; they are created in the liver from excess sugars the body has not used for energy. These sugars come from refined sugar, boxed cereal, white flour, and other foods containing processed, refined carbohydrates.

Take notice—when you partake in these processed foods you feel tired, weighed down, bloated, and sluggish.

CHAPTER TEN

We Took the Fat Out
of the American Diet,
and We Got Fatter and Sicker

*...Come unto me: and I will give you the good of the land
of Egypt, and ye shall eat the fat of the land.*
—Genesis 45:18 KJV

Before we talk about oils, let's first talk about the different types
of fat. We've learned to be terrified of fat, even though taking
the fat out of the American diet made us fatter and sicker. Heart
disease is the leading cause of death in the United States. Bone
loss, reduction in height, and brain and neurological disorders
are on the rise due to removing healthy fats from the diet and
replacing them with processed oils known as *trans fats*.

What Exactly is Fat?

Fat is made up of a carbon atom that is measured in different
lengths of chains. Some fats have short chains of carbon

atoms, some have medium, some have longer chains, and some have extra-long chains. Yes, there are good fats and bad fats. Removing the good fats from your diet can be extremely unhealthy, causing a laundry list of serious health conditions. The good news is that there is not a bad fat found in nature.

Saturated Fats

Fatty acids are *saturated* when a hydrogen atom occupies all available carbon bonds. They are highly stable, because all the carbon-atom linkages are filled or saturated with hydrogen. This means that these fats do not normally go rancid, and they don't pose a health risk when cooked at higher temperatures. They liquefy with heat, and they form a solid or semisolid fat at room temperature.

Monounsaturated Fats

Monounsaturated fatty acids have two carbon atoms that are double-bonded to each other and, therefore, lack two hydrogen atoms. Your body makes monounsaturated fatty acids from saturated fatty acids and uses them in numerous ways. Monounsaturated fat molecules have a bend at the position of the double bond so that they do not pack together as easily as saturated fats do; therefore, they are liquid at room temperature. Like saturated fats, they are relatively stable. Monounsaturated fats do not go rancid easily. They are heat stable and therefore very good for cooking and baking. The monounsaturated fat most commonly found in our food is oleic acid, the main component in nuts, olive oil, and avocados.

Polyunsaturated

Polyunsaturated fatty acids have about four double bonds that lack four or more hydrogen atoms. The two polyunsaturated fatty acids found in our foods are double unsaturated linoleic acid, which have two double bonds — also called omega-6 — and triple unsaturated linoleic acid, with three double bonds.

The omega number indicates the position of the first double bond. Your body cannot make these fatty acids, and they are called *essential*. We must obtain our essential fatty acids — EFAs — from the foods we eat. They go rancid very quickly, particularly omega-3 linoleic acid, and must be treated with care.

Polyunsaturated fats are simply fat molecules that have more than one saturated carbon bond in the molecule, which is also called a double bond. Polyunsaturated fats are found in small amounts in green vegetables, grains, legumes, fish, nuts, and olive oil. The Standard American Diet (SAD) consists of high levels of polyunsaturated oils but in the form of hydrogenated oils, such as corn, canola, and soy. These oils are used in most prepackaged and processed foods as preservatives. They are the culprits of free radical damage, disorders of the brain, depressed learning ability, impaired growth, heart disease, and cancer. Now in my opinion, that's sad.

The bottom line is that you can have small amounts of polyunsaturated fats that are naturally occurring in most foods. However, you should avoid hydrogenated fats in the form of processed vegetable oils. *These oils should be avoided due to their detrimental health effects.*

What Is Hydrogenation?

Hydrogenation is a process that leads to trans fatty acids. Trans fats are unhealthy fats that form when vegetable oil hardens in a process called hydrogenation. Pumping hydrogen into the liquid oil at an extremely high temperature creates trans fats. These oils are also labeled *partly hydrogenated*. This process damages the molecules making them difficult to break down and digest.

Hydrogenated oils contribute to a laundry list of serious health conditions due to oxidization and rancidity when subjected to heat. Rancid oils are known to cause allergies, asthma, and other autoimmune-related diseases. Free radical damage occurs through oxidation which, in turn, causes damage to the immune system. Oxidation leads to accelerated cell damage, which produces wrinkles and premature aging of the skin, tissues, and organs. Theses circumstances set the stage for tumors and DNA damage.

THE RATIO OF OMEGA-3 VERSUS OMEGA-6

Too Much Omega-6

Excess consumption of these oils can result in:

- Increased blood clots
- Inflammation
- High blood pressure
- Cancer
- Heart disease
- Digestive complications
- Depressed immune function
- Infertility
- Cell proliferation

Too Little Omega–3

The Standard American Diet (SAD) is deficient in omega–3s, linoleic acid. Omega–3 acid is necessary for:

- Healthy cell formation
- Metabolizing the breakdown of food
- Maintaining proper balance in hormone production
- The prevention of cancer
- Heart health

Diets low in omega–3s have been associated with asthma, learning deficiencies, and heart disease. Omega–3 is a natural anti-inflammatory essential fatty acid.

Unfortunately, chicken, fish, and animals raised in feedlots feast on processed and genetically modified feed that contains too much omega–6 and virtually no omega–3. Pasture-raised eggs from hens allowed to feed on insects and green plants contain a perfect ratio of omega–3 and omega–6 of approximately one-to-one. This is unlike the commercial supermarket eggs and meats which can contain as much as twenty times more omega–6 than omega–3.

Consuming these inflammatory foods may lead to conditions such as:

- Cancer
- Heart disease
- Thyroid issues
- Autoimmune disorders
- Brain and neurological conditions

Now that you understand the connection between modern diets and modern diseases, let's talk about the benefits of fat that has been falsely vilified as the *bad fat* known as saturated fats.

The Benefits of Saturated Fats

Saturated fat plays critical roles in body chemistry. Saturated fatty acids constitute at least 50 percent of the cell membranes in the body. They are what give our cells necessary stiffness and integrity.

Saturated fats are some of the best fats for the heart. Yes, I did say that. The fat around the heart muscle is highly saturated. The heart draws on this reserve of fat especially in times of stress. Following all the saturated fat reduction hype has increased heart disease.

Saturated fat protects us against harmful microorganisms in the digestive tract. Saturated fat plays a vital role in the health of our bones. For calcium to be effectively incorporated into the skeletal structure, we need our diets to contain saturated fats daily. They lower lipoproteins, or LP(a)s. The short- and medium-chain fatty acids in saturated fat also have immune enhancing antimicrobial properties.

It doesn't end here; saturated fats protect the liver from toxins. They support the immune system. So in my opinion—and now hopefully yours—*artery-clogging* saturated fats causing heart disease is a myth.

Oils

So now that you understand the composition of fats, let's talk about the best oils for cooking as well as drizzling on cold dishes and smoothies.

The best oils are called *extra-virgin*, which are cold-pressed, a chemical-free process that involves only cold pressure leaving the oil with optimal flavor and highest nutritional value.

Olive Oil

Extra virgin olive oil is high in monounsaturated fats and contains generous amounts of vitamins E and K2 of the fat-soluble vitamins.

Extra virgin olive oil is loaded with antioxidants, which have many powerful health benefits. It contains anti-inflammatory properties, such as oleic acid, and when consumed may positively impact:

- Heart disease
- Cancer
- Metabolic syndrome
- Diabetes
- Alzheimer's disease
- Arthritis

Olive oil may be one of the healthiest foods for your heart. It lowers blood pressure, protects cells from oxidation, and may help prevent unwanted blood clotting. Olive oil is best for cold dishes as this oil has longer chains of carbon atoms, making olive oil not very heat stable.

What does *refined* mean?

Refined means that the nutrients have been removed through damaging processes such as bleaching, milling, and deodorizing, causing the product to be less nutritious.

The Different Varieties of Olive Oil

Kelly Martinez, managing director of the Antonion Celetano olive oil company in Spain, explains the classifications of olive oil:

Olive oil is olive juice. *Virgin oil,* according to Martinez, is a label meaning "mechanical extraction." Machines extract the oil or juice with no chemicals used in the process. (Martinez, 2005)

Mechanically extracted (virgin) olive oil has different levels of quality. *Extra* is the label used for the highest quality because this oil goes through laboratory and taste tests. When the olives are first pressed to extract the oil, the initial pressing produces the richest tasting oil. Extra virgin olive oil is best for salad dressings and drizzling on food just before its served. Perform your own taste test!

Olive oil with slight defects that is still good for human consumption is classified as *fine.*

Low quality oil with numerous defects is classified as either *ordinary* or *lampante* (lamp oil). This oil is either used for industrial purposes or is chemically refined. In other words, ordinary olive oil is refined oil that has most likely been bleached and deodorized, creating an odorless, colorless, and tasteless oil. I would suggest that you avoid this oil at all costs.

Olive oil that is not suitable for human consumption is refined by a heat and chemical process. Refined oils in general are oxidized by the heat of processing. Heat denatures and damages the vital nutrients. Chemically refined oil is flavorless and low quality. Refined oil is mixed with virgin oil for color and flavor (Martinez, 2005). It is not a wise choice.

Be Aware of Oil Blends

Pomace oil is made from the waste of virgin olive oil after the oil is extracted. High heat and chemicals produce an oil that is flavorless and meets no quality standards. Pomace oil is mixed with virgin oil so that it has flavor. Not a wise choice.

Some oils are labeled *pure, light,* or *extra light.* They are blends of lower quality oil with virgin oil. Mixes — or blends as packers like to call them — are generally 90–95 percent pomace and refined virgin oil. Some packers mix in seed, or soy oil, which cheapens the cost (Martinez, 2005).

Also note that *light* olive oil does not mean lower in calories. All olive oils have the same number of calories, so please don't fall for these marketing strategies when buying oil.

Refined oil and virgin oil are *not the same.* Refined oil mixes are cheap to produce and cheaper to buy than quality oils. They are marketed with deceiving strategies, leading you to believe they are better for you, and therefore these mixes benefit the seller more than you and me.

How to Store Olive Oil

You do not need to refrigerate olive oil. Refrigerating or freezing does not harm any type of olive oil, but it will thicken it. You'll have to let it come to room temperature so it is pourable again. According to the International Olive Oil Council, olive oil expands about 2 to 4 percent with refrigeration or freezing and may shatter the glass bottle.

Store your olive oil in a closed container, away from heat or light. A good quality extra virgin olive oil has a shelf life of twelve to eighteen months. Keep your olive oil in a dark spot for storage, preferably in your pantry. Avoid direct exposure to sunlight.

Olive Oil History

The olive tree is native to the Mediterranean basin. The olive is a subtropical, broad-leaved, perennial tree. Archaeological records indicate olives have been eaten for more than thirty thousand years, and that humans have cultivated the tree for at least six thousand years (MDidea Extracts, 2014).

The olive tree ranges in height from 10 to 40 feet or more and can attain a great age. Some trees in the eastern Mediterranean are estimated to be more than two thousand years old. Olives originated in Asia Minor and in Ancient Greece and about six thousand years ago, spread along the coasts of the Mediterranean between the thirtieth and forty-fifth parallels.

The best sources for olive oil are in the resource section of this book.

Coconut Oil

There are essentially two types of coconut oil—*virgin* and *refined*. Pressing fresh coconut meat, coconut milk, or coconut milk residue releases virgin coconut oil, or VCO.

Refined, bleached, and deodorized coconut oil is made from the coconut *copra* or dried kernel and may be chemically treated. This is not a healthy food choice.

Telling the Difference

Virgin coconut oil and refined coconut oils both have the same milky white appearance. Therefore, appearance only cannot distinguish between the two.

Virgin coconut oil tastes and smells like coconut, while refined coconut oil is essentially free of odor and flavor. It is also free of much of the nutritive value of VCO, making refined coconut oil an unhealthy choice.

Unlike olive oil, there isn't much difference between virgin or *extra* virgin coconut oil. Both virgin and extra virgin coconut oil are cold-pressed from fresh mature coconuts with no heat, deodorizers, or bleaching agents applied.

Both virgin and extra virgin coconut oil contain medium-chain essential fatty acids, which are the shorter chains of carbon atoms. Coconut oil is highly heat stable, which makes it an excellent choice for cooking and baking. This oil retains all its enzymes and nutrients during the heating process and does not create rancidity.

Lauric Acid

Coconut oil is high in *lauric* acid, essential for preventing unfriendly bacteria or microbes in the gut. Lauric acid accounts for 50 percent of the fatty acids present in coconut oil having the potential to kill harmful pathogens.

The human body converts lauric acid into *monolaurin*, which is beneficial in combatting viruses and bacteria that cause diseases such as herpes and influenza. Monolaurin also fights other harmful bacteria present in the digestive tract that lead to disease. Coconut oil destroys pathogens that are active in the blood.

Coconut oil has tremendous antimicrobial properties. It is antifungal, antiviral, and anti-Candida. Coconut oil has also played a role in the reversal of colds and flus.

HEALTH BENEFITS OF COCONUT OIL

Heart Health

Coconut oil contains large quantities of saturated fats and has therefore gained a bad reputation of being unhealthy for the heart. Coconut oil is beneficial for the heart. The saturated fats present in coconut oil are not harmful like the fats found in refined vegetable oils. Despite the misinformation about saturated fats and coconut oil, it reduces the incidence of damage to arteries and therefore helps prevent hardening of the arteries or arteriosclerosis.

Skin Care

Coconut oil is an excellent massage oil as well as a great remedy for dry skin. It also delays the appearance of wrinkles and sagging of skin. I have found that coconut oil helps in successfully treating various skin problems including psoriasis, eczema, and dermatitis. Coconut oil is a base ingredient for various body care products like soaps, lotions, toothpaste, and deodorant. I use coconut oil every day in skin, hair, and body care products. Coconut oil also helps prevent accelerated aging due to its high antioxidant properties.

The Fat That Makes You Lose Fat

Coconut oil is widely used today because it contains short- and medium-chain fatty acids that help shed those excess pounds. More than 90 percent of coconut oil consists of saturated fat, true. Don't panic; remember the benefits of saturated fat.

The medium-chain fatty acids in coconut oil help balance the metabolism and regulate digestion by increasing the body's metabolic rate. This process removes stress on the pancreas and liver, the organs needed for optimal digestion. The pancreas and liver are the two organs that excrete enzymes necessary for digestion, and enzymes are catalysts that help break down fats, proteins, and carbohydrates. The saturated fat in coconut oil keeps you feeling full for a longer time and sustains your body. The calories that are provided by the fat in coconut oil are converted into energy approximately fifteen minutes after consumption.

Coconut oil is a number-one fuel for the thyroid and endocrine system. Coconut oil helps burn more energy while helping lose unwanted weight. People who use coconut oil every day as their primary cooking oil express healthy weight and have little to no incidences of thyroid issues. Coconut oil is also rich in omega–3 essential fatty acids, a naturally occurring anti-inflammatory.

Saturated Fatty Acid

Saturated fats are medium-chain triglycerides containing single bonds of carbon atoms which assimilate extremely well into the body's systems. Lauric acid, capric acid, caprylic acid, and myristic acid are all known to reduce inflammation in the body that contributes to disease.

Polyunsaturated fatty acid is also known as linoleic acid.

Monounsaturated fatty acid is also known as oleic acid.

Present in coconut oil are *polyphenols*, compounds that contain more than one group of *phenolic hydroxyl*, an organic chemistry of compounds. Coconut contains *gallic acid*, which is also known as *phenolic acid*. These polyphenols are responsible for the wonderful coconut scent and the delicious taste. Phenolic hydroxyl and phenolic acid are beneficial to the human body due to their antioxidant properties. Antioxidants have the ability to fight against free radical damage.

These critical healing benefits make coconut oil a wise choice for cooking, baking, and care of skin, hair, and body—inside and out.

How to Store Coconut Oil

Coconut oil is shelf stable for up to two years. Depending on the indoor temperature and the season, this could mean it is either a liquid or a solid, depending on the temperature. I am not a fan of storing coconut oil in the refrigerator, because it will be hard and more difficult to use. Storing your coconut oil in the pantry is best and will not affect its quality or shorten the shelf life.

A Brief History of Coconut Oil

The term *coconut* derives from the sixteenth century Spanish and Portuguese words *coco*, meaning monkey face. The coconut has a hairy shell and resembles the face of a monkey. The coconut is considered a fruit; however, this fruit consists of three layers which is a called a drupe. These layers are called the *exocarp*, *mesocarp*, and the *endocarp*. The exocarp and endocarp represent the husk of the fruit. The mesocarp contains a seed fiber. The mesocarp is used to produce brushes, ropes, and fishnets.

For the past four thousand years, the fruits of the coconut palm have been used both as food and medicine. Coconut oil has sustained the lives of tropical communities. This popular staple of coconut flesh, water, milk, and oil richly benefited many.

Many tropical regions around the world use coconut oil:

- South America
- Central America
- Africa
- Indian subcontinent
- Polynesia
- Asia

In 1500 BCE, the uses of coconut oil were documented in Ayurvedic medicine.

Early European explorers wrote about the multiple medicinal benefits of using coconut oil every day. During World War I, young green coconut water was substituted for saline drips, saving lives and extending exhausted supplies. After the war, coconut oil was sold as a butter replacement in England and as coconut butter in the United States (Marson, 2014). Incorporating coconut oil into your diet is a wise choice. Be sure to use organic, extra virgin or virgin coconut oil for optimal taste and nutritional value.

The best coconut oil sources can be found in the resource section of this book.

Palm Oil

Palm oil comes from a tropical tree. *Virgin palm oil* is known for its high antioxidants. Beware of the refined versions, which are bleached and deodorized, resulting in an oil stripped of nutrients and clear in color. In its natural state, palm oil is red in color due to a high concentration of carotenes and tocols.

Palm oil, similar to coconut oil, has traditionally been used in cooking and baking because it is heat stable. This oil solidifies at room temperature and liquefies during heating without losing vital nutrients.

Certified, Sustainable Palm Oil

Recently, the use of palm oil has come under criticism because of the deforestation necessary to grow palm tree farms. Certified sustainable palm oil (CSPO) is oil that has grown on plantations managed and certified by the Roundtable on Sustainable Palm Oil (RSPO). Certification by RSPO means that the plantation was established on land that did not contain significant biodiversity, wildlife habitat, or any other environmental values. CSPO also represents palm oil that meets the highest environmental, economic, and social standards, as set out by the RSPO.

The RSPO was established in 2004 to promote the production of sustainable palm oil for the planet, people, and prosperity. Choose Certified Sustainable Palm Oil—the highest quality of palm oil. CSPO will have a seal on the label that reads Certified Sustainable Palm Oil RSPO.

Benefits of Palm Oil

In nature, there are approximately six hundred known carotenoids. They range in color from red to orange to yellow. Approximately fifty of these pigments contain some degree of vitamin A. Palm oil receives its reddish color from the carotenes beta-carotene and lycopene, the same nutrients that give carrots and tomatoes their pigment. The oil of red palm contains the phytonutrients tocotrienols (vitamin E), mixed carotenoids, phytosterols, squalene, and coenzyme Q10 (CoQ10).

These vital nutrients are proven to support both cardiovascular and neurological health. Virgin palm oil is one of the richest natural plant sources of these carotenoids. It has twenty times more carotenoids than carrots and three hundred times more than tomatoes. No other vegetable oil contains carotenoids in such substantial amounts. I am a bigger fan of coconut oil for cooking and smoothies due to its rich coconut taste; however; organic, unrefined, virgin red palm oil is a fantastic cooking oil due to its high heat stability.

Be sure that your palm oil is organic, unrefined, and red in color to ensure that bleaching agents were not used in the processing. Palm kernel oil does not convey the same health benefits as red palm oil, but does not pose any health dangers when used in smaller quantities.

Palm oil can be sold fresh or oxidized. Oxidation results when the oil is processed for various culinary purposes. However, a considerable amount of palm oil on the market is in the oxidized state, which poses potential dangers to the biochemical and physiological functions of the body (Axe, 2014). Unlike fresh, unrefined palm oil, oxidized palm oil damages the lipid profile, creating reproductive toxicity of the kidney, lung, liver, and heart. Oxidized palm oil is also deodorized and bleached, turning the oil white. I highly suggest that you never use colorless palm oil as this is not what nature created.

History of Palm Oil

The history of palm oil originated five thousand years ago in West Africa, where palm oil was used as a staple food crop. Egyptian tombs reveal people buried with casks of palm oil, reflecting the value placed on it by the society. Palm oil was considered one of the earliest traded commodities, and it is believed that Arab traders brought the oil to Egypt.

Palm oil is a common cooking ingredient in the tropical areas of Africa, Asia, and in some parts of Brazil. Palm oil is used in many recipes for cooking and baking worldwide due to its inexpensive price.

Red palm oil is another healthy, wise choice.

Walnut Oil

Walnut oil is extracted from English walnuts, also known as Persian walnuts. Each 100 grams of oil provides about 63.3 grams of polyunsaturated fatty acids, 22.8 grams of monounsaturated fats, and 9.1 grams of saturated fats. It contains no cholesterol.

Unlike other nut oils, unrefined walnut oil is made from nuts that are dried first and then cold-pressed. Its flavor is rich and nutty, perfect for salad dressings or drizzling over your favorite dishes. Walnut oil is not only wonderful for drizzling, but its rich, creamy, sweet taste is lovely to add to your favorite desserts. Walnut oil is best used uncooked or in cold dishes because when it is heated, it can become slightly bitter. However, some find the bitter taste pleasant when used in smaller quantities.

Walnut oil is extremely high in antioxidants that help fight the effects of aging. It is an excellent source of omega-3 fatty acids, which are essential fatty acids that the body needs for repair. The topical use of walnut oil helps reduce the appearance of fine lines and wrinkles. Walnut oil is great for massage and aromatherapy as well.

This versatile oil has many nutritional benefits and is loaded with anticancer compounds. This can be attributed to the high omega-3 fatty acids and other phytonutrients in walnut oil like *ellagitannins*.

Some of the benefits of walnut oil are as follows:

- Rich in antioxidants
- Great for weight loss
- Protects and polishes wood
- Antibacterial and antiviral agent on open wounds
- Strong anti-inflammatory (omega-3)
- Strong antifungal (protects against candida in the gut)
- Promotes regularity
- Anti-aging, especially on skin

History of Walnut Oil

Historical evidence has shown that walnuts have been in existence for thousands of years. Walnut oil has been used for a variety of purposes which included use as a holy oil. Walnuts were introduced to Europe through the Mediterranean. In isolated northern Italy, walnut oil was valued for flavor and usefulness.

The walnut crop was important in the Middle Ages. Officials punished those who snuck into groves to pick up fallen walnuts and imposed transport duties upon both walnuts and walnut oils. Walnuts were dried, shelled, and ground; the nut flour was then pressed to extract the oil. The making of walnut oil was a community activity, with families or neighborhoods helping each other work through their stands of trees.

Peanut Oil

Peanut oil is a sweet, flavorful, and edible oil obtained from pressing fresh peanut kernels. Peanut oil is also known as *groundnut oil* which gets its name from *Arachis hypogea*, a low-growing, annual plant. Despite the word *nut* in its name, the peanut is a legume that grows underground. Other true nuts, like walnuts and almonds, grow on trees.

Peanut oil originated in South America. It eventually reached North America, Asia, and Africa by way of European explorers who brought it back to their own countries where peanuts were cultivated. Today, the top three producers of peanut oil are India, China, and the United States. Peanut oil is heat stable, making it safe for cooking.

The Problem with Peanut Oil

Peanuts are extremely high in omega-6 and therefore can be inflammatory when consumed in large amounts. Despite the many uses of peanut oil, it may not be safe for everybody. Peanuts contain allergens that account for a majority of severe food-related allergic reactions. Having a peanut allergy can be a serious and scary situation.

Symptoms of a peanut allergy may include:

- Runny nose
- Skin reactions — hives, redness, or swelling
- Digestive issues — diarrhea, cramping, nausea, or vomiting
- Tightening, itching, or tingling of the mouth or throat
- Shortness of breath, wheezing
- Death

Anaphylaxis is an acute allergic reaction and sometimes a deadly side effect of peanut oil. If you believe that you or someone you know may be having any of these symptoms after ingesting peanuts, seek immediate emergency attention as this can be fatal.

Peanut oil may be used in very small quantities and must be organic and unrefined to avoid genetic mutations and oxidation.

An Important Side Note on Peanuts

Peanuts contain a carcinogen called *aflatoxin*. This toxin is a poisonous, anti-nutrient known to cause liver cancer in rats and presumably in humans. This toxin is caused by mold to which peanuts are highly susceptible since they grow in warm, humid silos. This toxin is also present in organic peanuts and peanut butter, but not as potent. If you must indulge in peanuts, choose roasted, organic peanuts. The roasting process does eliminate most of the aflatoxin.

My best suggestion for peanuts that do not contain this carcinogen at all are wild jungle peanuts, which are a highly nutritious peanut and superfood. Jungle peanuts are high in omega-3, making them an anti-inflammatory food.

Almond Oil

The almond is a species of tree that is native to the Middle East and South Asia. *Almond* is also the name of the edible and widely cultivated seed of this tree. Oil from the almond can be made into almond milk and almond butter, two of my personal favorites.

Almond oil is one of the richest oils for hair and skin care. It is packed with nutrients and beneficial properties, which make it such a powerful cosmetic ingredient. The results obtained by using almond oil on skin and hair can be compared to many powerful beauty care products, without all the unnecessary side effects. Applying a small amount of almond oil under your eyes can help minimize the appearance of dark circles.

There are many varieties of almonds, but they are generally classified into two categories: bitter almonds and sweet almonds.

Bitter Almonds

Bitter almonds produce bitter almond oil which is banned in the United States. These almonds are hardly ever eaten or used in recipes. Not only do they have an unpleasant taste, but these almonds contain a small amount of *hydrogen cyanide*, which is extremely poisonous. Bitter almonds contain glycoside amygdalin which turns into prussic acid, or hydrogen cyanide, when consumed.

Cyanide was the key ingredient used in Nazi gas chambers. Eating just a few of these almonds can lead to severe dizziness, vertigo, or even death. If you are hiking in the woods and come across an almond tree, please don't assume that it is safe to partake in these nuts. A few handfuls of bitter almonds have the potential to kill you, consuming just a few can cause serious health issues that can lead to kidney failure.

I would hope you avoid bitter almonds now that you've learned their bitter truth.

Sweet Almonds

Sweet almonds are different than bitter almonds. Yes, these are the almonds that we are accustomed to eating. These almonds are used to produce sweet almond oil, which is delicious and perfectly safe to eat. Sweet almonds—including their oil—are extremely effective in optimizing digestion and colon heath. Consumption of this oil reduces the risk of developing rectal and colon cancer.

Drinking almond oil may delay or even stop the conversion of benign and cancerous polyps. Almond oil applied directly on the skin minimizes the appearance of scarring. This also applies to stretch marks, dry skin, psoriasis, and eczema. I have recommended the topical use of sweet almond oil to patients suffering from various skin conditions and have seen positive results. This is attributed to the high antioxidant properties found in the oil.

All nut oils are fragile and best used unheated to retain the most antioxidants, vitamins, and flavor. Therefore, almond oil is great for cold dishes, salads, and smoothies. Almond oil is also quite lovely in low-heat cooking. As with all oils, almond oil should always be organic and unrefined to avoid chemical fertilizers and oxidation that can be dangerous to our health.

A Natural Headache Remedy

Almonds contain a natural pain-reducing compound called *salicin*. This is the same ingredient found in aspirin without the harmful side effects. Enjoy a handful or two of almonds—about fourteen almonds—and start reducing your pain. Almonds may be a triggering food for migraines; however, that may be due to having been roasted in rancid oils.

Sesame Oil

Sesame seeds have been in use for more than five thousand years. These amazing seeds are one of the most nutrient-rich, powerhouse foods on the planet. These seeds are also valued for their rancid-resistant oil.

In fact, once you learn of the many health benefits of this ancient condiment, you will want to stock up your pantry with this oil.

The health benefits of sesame oil include:

- Promotes heart health/helps reduce blood pressure
- Protects against radiation and chemotherapy-induced DNA damage
- Helps restore and rebuild bone mineral density
- Alleviates iron deficiency anemia
- Promotes healthy skin
- Helps prevent headaches and migraines
- Reduces stress
- Regulates hormones
- Prevents constipation
- Stabilizes blood glucose levels in diabetics

Sesame Oil as Food

Sesame oil has a strong flavor and complements the taste of Asian and stir-fry recipes. This oil is also nice in salads when you're looking for an Asian flair. If you use sesame oil for cooking, the fragrant sesame aroma will stimulate your appetite. Just the right amount, a small amount that is, adds a heavenly, nutty flavor to Asian dishes.

Now you know that sesame oil is the hidden, healthy ingredient in most Asian dishes.

Tonijean's Easy Organic Asian Sauce Recipe

In a bowl combine:
½ cup organic coconut garlic teriyaki by Coconut Secret — find at coconutsecret.com
½ cup organic, toasted sesame oil

Mix well.

This simple sauce can be poured over steamed veggies or a salad for an Asian taste. This recipe is suitable for 2 cups steamed veggies or 2 ½ cups of mixed raw salad veggies. Double the recipe ingredients for larger dishes. Yummo!

There are multiple varieties of sesame oil today as well as variations in color. Cold-pressed sesame oil is pale yellow while Indian sesame oil is golden, and East Asian sesame oils are usually a dark brown in color. The dark color and flavor are derived from roasted or toasted sesame seeds. Cold-pressed sesame oil has a different flavor than the toasted oil since it is produced directly from raw, rather than toasted seeds. Cold-pressed sesame oil is available in most health food stores or online. Unroasted—but not necessarily cold-pressed—sesame oil is commonly used for cooking in Middle East markets. In East Asian countries, different kinds of hot-pressed sesame oil are often preferred.

Sesame oil has gained its popularity for its unique flavor as well as its high antioxidant content. There are high amounts of fat-soluble vitamin E found in sesame oil that are retained in the oil when it is cold-pressed. Once again, I suggest that any product including sesame oil be organic for optimal flavor and nutritional value.

Sources of peanut, walnut, sesame, and sweet almond oil can be found in the resource section of this book.

Hemp Seed Oil

Hemp oil or hemp seed oil is obtained by pressing hemp seeds. Cold-pressed, unrefined hemp oil is dark to clear, light green in color, with a nutty flavor. The darker the color, the better the flavor and nutritional value. Hemp seed oil is great for drizzling on food as well as adding to smoothies. This oil is not heat stable, so it is not a good choice for cooking.

Hemp seed oil has a 3:1 ratio of omega-6 to omega-3 fatty acids, a balance known to be beneficial for cardiovascular health. Hemp seed oil is among one of the most widely used oils in the holistic industry. It's high omega-3 content makes this oil attractive due to its anti-inflammatory properties.

The properties of hemp seed oil may protect against the aging process. Hemp seed oil contains essential fatty acids, including *docosahexaenoic acid* (DHA), which is needed for brain development. DHA is also critical for the health of the retina of the eyes.

Another antioxidant in hempseed oil is *tocopherol*, which is beneficial against degenerative diseases such as heart disease, arthritis, dementia, and Alzheimer's. Hemp seed oil is loaded with anticancer elements. It may also be an excellent medicine for the reversal of cancerous tumors.

Hemp seed also has high levels of vitamins A, C, and E and is rich in minerals like phosphorus, potassium, calcium, magnesium, and sulfur. In addition, it tastes great.

History of Hemp Seed Oil

A derivative of *cannabis* or marijuana, hemp has been used across the centuries in medicine, textiles, and food by people all over the world. Hemp is one of the oldest agricultural crops cultivated, dating back as early as 400 BCE in China.

Hemp is a term used for high-growing varieties of the cannabis plant. Its products include fiber, oil, and seed. The uses of the cannabis plant are innumerable, as it is made into products such as hemp seed, hemp oil, wax, resin, rope, cloth, pulp, paper, and fuel.

Hemp seed oil should be organic, raw, and unrefined. I use hemp seed oil on salads and in smoothies.

Sources for the best hempseed oil can be found in the resource section at the back of this book.

Flaxseed Oil

Flaxseed oil comes from the seeds of the flax plant. Flax is unique because, traditionally, the seed has been used more than the oil. The seed has been used whole, cracked, or ground into flour so it can be included in baked products.

Flaxseeds are nutritionally unique for their broad spectrum of nutrients such as calcium, magnesium, potassium, fiber, and omega-3 essential fatty acids. Flaxseed oil is high in *lignans*, which are high in antioxidant properties.

Flaxseeds can be sprinkled on oatmeal, salads, added to smoothies, and juiced. Use ground flaxseeds as the body cannot breakdown whole flaxseeds; they pass through the body undigested. Then you will miss out on all their wonderful benefits.

Flaxseed oil is high in the essential fatty acids omega-3, *alpha-linoleic acid* (ALA), *eicosapentaenoic acid* (EPA), and *docosahexaenoic acid* (DHA). Once consumed, the human body converts ALA to EPA and DHA, which are more readily used by the body.

History of Flaxseed Oil

Flaxseed is also known as linseed, *Linum usitatissimum*. Now that's a mouthful. It is a member of the genus *Linum* in the family *Lanaceae*. Flax has been cultivated for more than seven thousand years. The plant's brown seeds were regularly used to prepare balms for inflamed skin and as healing remedies for constipation.

Today, flaxseeds are best known for the therapeutic oil that is derived by pressing the seeds. Flaxseed oil has earned a great reputation for treating a range of ailments ranging from heart disease, cancer, brain and neurological disorders to Lupus. Flaxseed oil has been used successfully as part of the holistic, healing protocol for cancer patients. Flaxseed oil is used to prevent and treat heart disease and to relieve a variety of inflammatory disorders and hormone-related problems, including infertility.

Flaxseed oil is an excellent source of omega-3 rich oil for cold dishes or drizzling. It is not a wise choice for cooking due to its inability to tolerate heat.

Sources of the best flaxseed oil can be found in the resource section of this book.

Avocado Oil

Avocados make a wonderful cooking oil due to high heat stability. Consumption of avocados makes it easy to shed those unwanted pounds. Avocados and avocado oil are high in monounsaturated oleic acid, a heart-healthy fatty acid compound. This may sound too good to be true, but avocados also have high fiber content, which is an additional health benefit. Fiber is indigestible plant matter that can contribute to weight loss, reduce blood sugar issues, and sustain you longer by making you fuller quicker. Fiber feeds the friendly gut bacteria in the intestine, which are important for the optimal function of our immune system. I consume an avocado daily, and if the avocado is larger in size, then I halve it. I encourage my patients to do the same.

History of Avocados

Avocados are a native fruit of South Central Mexico and have long been part of the Mexican diet. Avocado consumption dates as far as ten thousand years ago. Humans gathered wild avocados for their food and began cultivating them around five thousand years ago. The Incans and the Mesoamericans grew domesticated avocado trees. At the beginning of the seventeenth century, avocados began to receive serious attention from the United States. There was a wide difference of opinion for a name for this fruit, with almost forty different ideas. *Alligator pear* was considerably accepted by California and Florida, but horticulturists felt the name was a mistake, misleading, and ungraceful. The name "avocado" was approved by The American Pomological Society and the U.S. Department of Agriculture in the early 1900s.

Sources of avocado oil can be found in the resource section of this book.

The Oils Killing America

The following unnatural, manufactured vegetable fats and oils have the potential to cause serious digestive issues, thyroid malfunction, heart disease, immune system disorders, sterility, learning disabilities, growth problems, osteoporosis, and cancer:

- All hydrogenated oils (trans fats)
- Soy, corn, sunflower, and safflower oils

- Cottonseed oil
- Soybean oil
- Canola oil

The problem with these oils is the imbalance of omega–3 to omega–6 essential fatty acids (EFAs). The ratio of omega-3 and omega-6 in these oils is one to twenty. This lack of proportion creates an imbalance that can interfere with the production of important prostaglandins (fats) in the body. Consumption of these oils creates inflammation that eventually leads to disease.

Let's examine these oils and why they may be harmful.

Sunflower Oil

Sunflower oil is the nonvolatile oil made from pressing sunflower seeds. Sunflower oil is most commonly used as a frying oil for fast food and in prepackaged and processed foods. Sunflower oil is also used in cosmetic formulations as a skin moisturizer.

Why should sunflower oil be avoided?

All sunflowers oils are not alike: oil that is not expeller-pressed can be partially hydrogenated, which means it is high in trans fats and can increase your risk of heart disease and stroke. Hydrogenated oils are oxidized; therefore, I consider them damaged and artificial.

I hope you do not use this oil. It exacerbates inflammation in your body and puts you at risk for chronic diseases. Be aware of most prepackaged foods as they usually contain sunflower oil, making that food more inflammatory as well. Even some organic, prepackaged foods may contain sunflower oil as a preservative. Beware.

Safflower Oil

The safflower plant is a member of the sunflower family. It is an annual crop native to the Mediterranean, India, parts of Asia, and Africa. The use of safflower dates back more than five thousand years. Today, much of the Southwest, including California and Arizona, are home to the safflower crop.

History of Safflower Oil

Safflower is an orange-flowered, thistle-like Eurasian plant with seeds that yield edible oil; its petals were formerly used to produce red or yellow dyes. The wild safflower is native to North America; however, the plant cultivation took place in Russia. Safflower oil was first industrially produced in 1835 in the Russian Empire. It was only recently that the plant become a cultivated plant crop in the United States.

Cottonseed Oil

Cottonseed oil is extracted from the seeds of cotton plants of various species and is also known as a genetically modified crop.

Cottonseed oil is a common ingredient in many processed foods and animal feed and is widely used in restaurants as a cheap cooking oil for your favorite dishes, but I would not recommend it as part of your diet.

Cottonseed oil is by far one of the worst oils you can use. Poisons like *propargite, dicofol, cyanide*, and *trifluralin* are used on cotton to keep it safe from predators. When administered to cotton plants, these highly dangerous pesticides don't just stay on the surface, they absorb deep within the tissues, making cottonseed a highly toxic plant.

Cottonseed oil is a flavored ingredient in most breads, cereals, cookies, commercial salad dressings, and margarine. Once again, this oil is high in omega-6 with little to no omega-3, which means this oil is an inflammatory time bomb. This cheap oil is also hydrogenated with similar disease-forming compounds such as sunflower oil.

The Dirty Little Secret About Margarine and Vegetable Oils

Vegetable oils and margarine are oils extracted from seeds like corn, soybeans, and rapeseeds. They were nonexistent in our diets until the early 1900s when chemical processes were created that allowed them to be extracted.

Unlike butter or coconut oil, these oils cannot be extracted simply by cold-pressing or separating them naturally. They must be chemically removed, deodorized, and bleached, which contributes to their unhealthy qualities.

These oils are some of the most chemically altered foods in modern diets, yet they are promoted as health foods and sold in plastic tubs with deceiving marketing strategies in your local grocery stores.

Vegetable oils are found in every processed food on the market from salad dressing to butter substitutes to nut butters and prepackaged snacks. These oils are some of the most dangerous products you can put into your mouth.

Brace Yourself — How Vegetable Oils are Made

Vegetable oils are manufactured in factories using genetically modified crops that have been heavily treated with a ton of

We Took the Fat Out of the American Diet,
and We Got Fatter and Sicker
| 153

chemical fertilizers, which include pesticides, fungicides, and herbicides that are extremely detrimental to your health.

Canola Oil

Consider canola oil, the deceiving, so-called healthy oil of the vegetable oil industry. Everyone, including myself at one time, fell for this oil. It was given its name in the 1980s as part of a marketing strategy.

Rapeseed oil contains high amounts of the toxic *erucic acid*, which is heavily poisonous to the body. Canola oil is a genetically modified oil that does not exist in nature and is treated with high levels of chemical fertilizers. Rapeseeds, which are nonexistent in nature, are gathered to begin the canola process. Magnetized rods are used to remove any possible metal that may be present in the seeds. At this point, the canola is washed using *hexane*, a chemical compound used as a cleaning solvent. After the cleaning of the seeds is complete, a wash of *sodium hydroxide*, a corrosive substance, also known as *lye* and *caustic soda*, is then performed.

The last two processes include bleaching agents to lighten the cloudy product and steam injection to remove the potent smell. Then it is processed with a petroleum solvent to extract the oil. This removes the ugly-looking solids that form during the processing. Canola oil must then be treated with even more chemicals to improve the unpleasing grey color created while separating the different parts of the oil.

Here it is: this oil that must be chemically deodorized and bleached to make it taste, look, and smell pleasant.

You're probably wondering what the purpose of canola oil was in the first place. Canola oil was originally made to manufacture machinery and seal boats to protect them from weather-related issues. It is not fit for human consumption. Canola oil has been known to cause lesions on the heart due to its ability to deplete the body of magnesium and vitamin E, two important heart-healthy nutrients. Canola oil is commonly used in restaurants as the selected dressing oil drizzled on cold dishes.

Organic Canola Oil?

Canola, whether organic or not, still contains *glycosides*, a substance found in canola that inhibits enzyme production. Glycosides destroy the protective coating around the nerves or protective sheath. Glycosides are a form of sugar in which drugs and poisons are derived.

Canola consumption makes your body more vulnerable to heart disease, cancer, bronchial and respiratory conditions, emphysema, and anemia. All forms of canola, including organic varieties, are still deodorized at 300°F to remove the natural horrible odor. Even if farmers are not using chemical fertilizers on their *organic* canola plant, you are not out of the danger zone if you consume this oil.

Canola doesn't sound appetizing, does it?

Corn Oil

Corn oil is extracted from the germ of corn. Its main use is cooking; its high smoke point makes refined corn oil convenient for frying. It is also a cheap oil used in restaurants and fast food chains. It is one of the main ingredients in margarine. Corn oil comes from genetically modified crops, making this oil another dangerous choice.

Soybean Oil

Soybean oil is *not* a healthy oil. The majority of soybeans grown in the United States are genetically engineered, which contributes to many health conditions. Soybean oil is also hydrogenated, which makes it the worst type of oil you can put in your body.

The fat in soybean oil is primarily omega-6. It is rare for anyone to be deficient in omega-6, because it is so abundant in our diet. In general, most Americans consume too much omega-6. This overconsumption stems from the excessive amount of omega-6 found in processed foods, and animal foods raised on grain. The omega-6 fat in soy oil is highly processed and, therefore, damaged. This processing is a major contributor to oxidation that leads to accelerated aging and inflammatory diseases. The omega-6 found in soybean oil promotes chronic inflammation in your body, which is one of the main causes of all chronic diseases.

Organic Soybean Oil?

Even if you find organic soybean oil, it is far from being a healthy source of fat. Soy, whether organically grown or not, contains *goitrogens*, which are substances that block the synthesis of thyroid hormones and interfere with iodine metabolism and overall thyroid function. Soy consumption has been linked to digestive problems, thyroid dysfunction, cognitive decline, reproductive disorders, immune system breakdowns, heart disease, and cancer. Soy blocks the absorption of necessary minerals like calcium, magnesium, iron, and zinc, which get trapped in your intestines creating gas, bloating, and an extended belly. Soy oil, organic or not, is not a wise choice.

Shortening and Margarine

It's amazing how this chemically manufactured, toxic poison sitting on the grocery store shelf in big fat tubs is promoted as a *healthy* alternative to real butter, a God-made superfood.

When these vegetables oils are going to be made into shortening or margarine, they undergo an additional process called *hydrogenation* to make them solid at room temperature. Vegetable oils are not naturally solid at these temperatures and must be hydrogenated to make this process happen. During the hydrogenation process the dangerous trans fats begin to develop, making all vegetable oils refined, oxidized, poorly processed oils that are not wise choices.

Soybean, corn, and canola oils are commonly sold here in the United States and contain large amounts of trans fats. Trans fats are highly toxic poisons and major contributors to many diseases.

Why Are There so Many Reproductive Issues?

Vegetable oils in general are extremely damaging to the reproductive system, especially the body of a developing child. The dividing of cells during the reproduction process in the body can lead to cancer when these oils are consumed. You may be one of those people who at this point in your life have consumed tubs of margarine. You're most likely in a state of shock that you were led to believe the dreadful lie that butter and *saturated* fat are bad.

Avoiding canola, soy, and corn oil is a wise choice.

It's tough to learn the truthful dangers of some of the so called *healthy* oils and foods. You may have been consuming them thinking they are healthful sources for yourself and your family. The good news is that there are many delicious, highly nutritious oils that will not only compliment your food, but benefit your health.

Simply avoid using these trans fatty oils in your diet.

Knowing the truth will set you free from the bondage of sickness and the sick care industry.

Take a deep breath and congratulate yourself for completing the fats and oil section of this book.

CHAPTER ELEVEN

Farmed and Dangerous

What is the first thought that enters your mind when you think of eating fish?

It's healthy. Right?

A large variety of fish are packed with omega-3 essential fatty acids, rich in various types of nutrients and minerals, and high in an excellent source of protein.

So, is there a problem here? Well, depending on **the source** of your fish, you might be eating a host of antibiotic sewer sludge, or PCBs (*polychlorinated biphenyls*) that you're unaware of.

Sounds a little fishy now, doesn't it?

FARM RAISED OR WILD CAUGHT?

Farm Raised

Many health risks come with eating farmed fish. These fish are raised in commercial tanks, controlled pens, cesspools, and enclosures in estuaries, lakes, and ponds. These fish are not in their natural habitat where they have access to the abundance of the oceans' omega-3 rich foods provided by nature. Farmed fish are fed artificial and genetically modified pellet feed, loaded with toxins, artificial dyes, and antibiotics, and riddled with disease.

Does this sound like a healthy source of protein for your next dinner?

Farmed fish has an unbalanced ratio of omega-3 and omega-6. Consuming this source of fish puts us at a higher risk for inflammatory diseases, thyroid conditions, heart disease, arthritis, and certain types of cancers.

Ever wonder why wild-caught salmon has a much deeper orange-red color than farmed salmon?

This pigment is more than just a pretty color. It's a powerful antioxidant known to reduce inflammation, prevent cancer, stimulate the immune system, and is extremely beneficial in treating brain and neurological disorders. The deep-orange color is a result of *astaxanthin*, a naturally occurring carotenoid pigment found in microalgae, crustaceans, and wild fish such as salmon. Wild salmon feast on the abundance of the ocean, including crustaceans, algae, and krill.

Ever wonder how a flamingo gets its beautiful rosy pink color? The powerful antioxidant *astaxanthin*.

Farm-raised salmon consume a diet of artificially colored pellets to give them their distinctive pale pink color. A standard, farmed salmon chow contains soybean meal, corn gluten meal, poultry by-products, and canola meal.

Be aware of salmon labeled *Atlantic* and *Pacific*, as these are marketing terms that indicate the fish is farm-raised.

Wild Caught

Due to their natural diet, wild-caught fish tend to have much higher omega-3 essential fatty acids and protein than farmed fish. Wild fish is free from antibiotics, genetically engineered pellet feed, pesticides, and artificial dyes. They are free to roam about the ocean to find their own food. While mercury may be a small issue with some species of wild-caught fish, it can be so much more of an issue with farm-raised fish. Wild-caught fish contain an abundance of anti-inflammatory omega-3s and other nutrients, making it a far better choice.

I believe when it comes to consuming any food, our choices should be based on what the Creator has chosen for our consumption. The Almighty Physician is the Creator and knows best. Our first choice of fish should be wild with scales and fins, as described in scripture. As a believer of God's law, I recommend consuming only what He created for our food so we can enjoy great health.

> *These shall ye eat of all that are in the waters: whatsoever hath fins and scales in the waters, in the seas, and in the rivers, them shall ye eat. And all that have not fins and scales in the seas, and in the rivers, of all that move in the waters, and of any living thing which is in the waters, they shall be an abomination unto you.*
> — Leviticus 11:9-10 KJV

Catfish, lobsters, crabs, shrimp, mussels, clams, oysters, squid, and octopi are considered unclean because they are bottom feeders, which were created to clean up the ocean like little vacuum cleaners. When scientists test the water for mercury, they do not check fish that have scales and fins, because those fish expel toxins through their scales and fins. Scientists check the bottom feeders since they are the clean-up crew. The presence of these toxins in the tissues of bottom feeders creates inflammatory conditions and toxicity within your body when you consume them.

Why can fish consume crustaceans, yet the Bible says they are unclean?

The fish that dine on crustaceans are designed to play this role by nature. Fish of several species derive many benefits from eating shrimp and other shellfish and avoid any harmful effects that would be obtained by humans. Crustaceans are their natural diet just as the food we consume as humans may be beneficial to us, yet harmful to them. Live food including crustaceans for certain fish offers nutritional enhancement as well giving them their pigmentation.

Wild fish with scales and fins is exactly what you should fish for. Here is a list of Biblically clean healthy sources of fish:

- Cod
- Grouper
- Haddock
- Halibut
- Herring
- Mackerel
- Mahi Mahi
- Orange Roughy
- Pompano
- Trout
- Salmon
- Scrod
- Sea bass

- Snapper
- Sole
- Tuna
- Wahoo
- Whitefish

Once again be sure they are wild and not farmed.

Please take a break from reading and make a delicious wild flounder or wild cod dinner for your family. Here is my recipe.

Heat a stainless or cast iron skillet.

Add:
  1 heaping tablespoon of extra virgin coconut oil

Let oil melt on medium to low heat.

Add:
  2 cloves chopped organic garlic
  Sauté until lightly caramelized.

Add:
  2 pounds fresh, filleted wild cod or flounder
  Juice of 1 whole organic lemon
  Celtic sea salt
  Black pepper to your taste
  2 tablespoons organic butter

Allow the butter to melt. Flip the fish and cook the other side for 7 to 10 minutes, uncovered.

Add:
  ¼ cup fresh, chopped organic parsley

Cover with lid. Let steam on low heat until done—about 2 minutes.

Serve this wonderful dish with sweet potatoes, brown rice, or quinoa and a salad of choice.

The best wild fish sources can be found in the resource section of this book.

CHAPTER TWELVE

Don't Go Against the Grain

One of the most confusing topics in the health industry today is whether we should consume grains or avoid them. Unfortunately, many are led to believe that whole wheat breads and pasta are wise choices. In response to this marketing strategy and the many questions I receive about grains, I have written this chapter.

First, let's define a *grain*.

What is a grain?

Grains are any cultivated cereal crop used as food. Grains contain three parts—bran, endosperm, and germ—and the latter two are used as food.

All grains naturally have a special protection on them called *phytic acid* also called *anti-nutrients* or *enzyme inhibitors*. These naturally occurring antinutrients prevent the grain from being digested properly, resulting in gas, bloating, or a distended belly. These digestive symptoms are a result of nutrients becoming trapped in your intestines.

Inside the grain there are vital nutrients like fiber, minerals, and enzymes. However, for humans to absorb all the amazing benefits, the grains must be properly prepared through soaking or sprouting. We cannot benefit from the nutrients unless the phytic acid is broken down before we eat the grain.

Grains were consumed and enjoyed healthfully in biblical and ancient times. Today grains are being avoided due to the many health concerns that they cause. There are many health issues associated with modern grains from improper preparation, genetic engineering, chemical fertilizers, and enriching or fortifying with synthetic vitamins. Most packaged grains on the market contain ingredients that we can't even pronounce.

> *Take wheat and barley, beans and lentils, millet and spelt;*
> *put them in a storage jar and use them to make bread for*
> *yourself. You are to eat it during the 390 days you lie on*
> *your side.*
>
> —Ezekiel 4:9 NIV

Increasing Bioavailability

Germinating the grains through soaking or sprouting will remove the anti-nutrients and germinate the enzymes, vitamins, and minerals. I like to think of germinating as a process that brings the grain to life. This process makes the nutrients come alive, maximizing nutrient availability for optimal digestion and assimilation.

When you don't properly prepare grains before you consume them, they may even feel like a hard rock in your digestive tract. Phytic acid's job is to *hold on to the nutrients*; it won't release the fiber, nutrients, minerals, and enzymes your body needs. It will even steal nutrients from other food currently in your digestive tract.

Improperly prepared grains result in bloating, constipation, diarrhea, nutrient deficiencies, malabsorption, and eventually autoimmune conditions may occur. Gas and bloating are an indication that iron, calcium, magnesium, zinc, and copper have become trapped in your intestines and therefore your body can't use these nutrients properly.

By properly preparing grains you are basically breaking down the grain prior to ingesting it. This process signals the grain to open and release the *phytase*, which is the enzyme that breaks down phytic acid, making the nutrients in the grain more bioavailable for better assimilation.

Properly preparing the grain heightens the nutritional content of the grain and allows your body to absorb the nutrition the grain offers. The nutrients are now active and alive due to a soaking process called sprouting. Sprouting the grain resolves any tummy issues.

Sprouting?

The process of sprouting grains was used in ancient and biblical times. The process involves soaking the grains in water until they begin to grow. The grain becomes a live food, making it easier to assimilate the valuable nutrients. Enzymes are also released during the sprouting process. These enzymes break down proteins and carbohydrates and make them easier to digest.

Sprouting also lowers the glycemic value. The glycemic index indicates how quickly a food travels into your bloodstream and affects your blood glucose levels. Sprouted grains are suitable for diabetics and people with carbohydrate sensitivity, a condition resulting from consumption of modern, processed grains. Sprouted ancient grains have higher levels of protein and fiber, allowing the grain to enter the bloodstream slowly without the spike in blood sugar that occurs with improperly prepared grains.

The detrimental effects on the pancreas from the consumption of modern grains equal eating refined sugar directly out of the sugar bowl.

Most modern grain breads are difficult to digest, and therefore the body loses a large portion of the nutrients because it is unable to digest them. Sprouted grain breads provide the body with grain that has already been broken down, the enzymes and nutrients more available. Nutrients and minerals are absorbed immediately into the body and are not trapped in the intestines during the digestive process. The minerals zinc, calcium, magnesium, copper, and iron are now well assimilated and utilized by the body.

Germinating is a process that occurs during sprouting or soaking the grains, and releases all the vital nutrients stored in whole grains. I like to call germinating the process that predigests the grain by breaking down the nutrient content for easier digestion.

Beans and Gas?

First, let's define a *bean*. Beans are the common name for large seeds of the flowering plant family. Beans are edible seeds known as legumes, or leguminous plants that are used for human and animal food.

What's All the Gas About?

Beans or legumes contain a sugar called *oligosaccharide* that the body cannot break down. This undigested sugar results in gas. Therefore, beans also need to be soaked to make them digestible. Flatulence and bloating will ensue if the nutrients beans contain become trapped in your intestines. When minerals and nutrients cannot be assimilated properly in a grain, this is an indication that the grain has not been prepared properly through soaking. Lentils are also considered a bean that require soaking for better digestion.

How to Properly Soak Beans

Legumes, like grains, also contain phytic acid as well as enzyme inhibitors. Prior to cooking your beans, you must soak them in an acidic medium to remove these anti-nutrients including *oligosaccharides*. Kidney-shaped beans are soaked at the ration of one cup beans to two cups pure water, with a pinch of nonaluminum baking soda as the acid medium. They should soak in a pot for twelve to twenty-four hours. All beans, including lentils, require the same process except the acid medium is one tablespoon of lemon juice or raw apple cider vinegar instead of baking soda. For optimal digestibility, rinse and change the water and acid medium twice during the time of soaking. This process will deactivate the anti-nutrients and make the beneficial nutrients readily available.

Oatmeal

Most people I know love their oatmeal as their staple breakfast food but experience gas and bloating after a hearty bowl. Oats can be a highly nutritious grain, but they also require soaking for better assimilation. Oats also contain the protective coating phytase, or phytic acid.

Instant and Quick Oats

Oatmeal is available in many forms: instant, quick-cooking, old-fashioned, steel-cut, and whole oat groats. Unfortunately, the most popular form of oatmeal is instant oats, which may increase your risk of blood sugar imbalances, digestive issues, and heart disease due because they:

- Are lowest in soluble fiber
- Have the highest glycemic index
- Are sweetened with refined and artificial sugars
- Contain chemical-laden ingredients that are not real food

The glycemic index indicates how quickly a food travels into the bloodstream. The glycemic index chart runs from 0–100 indicating the affect carbohydrate-containing food has on blood glucose levels when consumed. Quick or instant oats have a glycemic load as high as 69 while regular, whole oats rank 55 or lower.

Why is soluble fiber important? Water-soluble fiber forms a gel within the digestive tract and provides many beneficial health effects. Oatmeal is high in soluble fiber (specifically *beta-glucan),* which increases excretion of bile acids.

Shopping for Oats

Organic rolled oats is another term for oatmeal, and they are what I use. Steel-cut oats or pinhead oatmeal are whole oat groats or hulled kernels, which have been chopped into pieces. Various forms of oatmeal, rolled oats, and pinhead oats are cooked to make porridge. If they are organic and soaked, they are highly nutritious as well as digestible.

By the way, oatmeal is naturally gluten free. What makes oats contain gluten is cross contamination in a processing plant.

Preparing Oats

Mix:
1 cup of organic rolled oats
1 cup of filtered or spring water
2 tablespoons plain, whole yogurt or buttermilk, lemon or apple cider vinegar

Cover with paper towel or dish towel overnight or for 8 hours. Do not refrigerate, as it is important for your oats to be in a warm kitchen or pantry. After they have soaked for the required time to remove the anti-nutrients, add:

1 additional cup of pure water
Real salt to taste

Simmer on medium heat for 4–5 minutes, stirring occasionally.

Serve with your favorite toppings.

You will feel more satisfied after eating properly prepared oats instead of unsoaked oats—no bloating, gas or discomfort. You will feel content from your hearty meal.

Nuts and Seeds

I love nuts and seeds. I consume them every day in the form of raw nut butters and whole as a crunchy snack. Nuts and seeds are a great way to add vitamins, minerals, fiber, and essential fatty acids for a healthy heart and brain to your diet. They are rich in minerals like magnesium and calcium—two critical nutrients for healthy bones and teeth. A few of the many great nuts include raw and organic almonds, pistachios, walnuts, cashews, pine nuts, macadamia, and Brazil nuts. Sesame, sunflower, hemp, flax, and chia are wonderful sources of seeds.

Nuts. A nut is a hard-shelled dry fruit or seed with a separable rind or shell and an interior, edible kernel. Nuts are a dry *indehiscent* — they don't open when ripe — with a woody *pericarp* as a kernel.

Seeds. A seed is "the grain or ripened ovules of plants used for sowing the fertilized ripened ovule of a flowering plant containing an embryo and capable normally of germination to produce a new plant" (Merriam-Webster, 2016).

Nuts and Seeds Will Keep You Regular

Nuts and seeds provide an excellent source of dietary fiber. Fiber is a specialized type of carbohydrate found in plant-based foods. Fiber adds bulk to your stool to promote regular bowel movements. Fiber also controls blood sugar levels by slowing down the rate of digestion. When fiber is present, the sugar from your food enters your bloodstream slowly, leading to a gradual increase in blood sugar. This gradual increase leaves you feeling energized after you eat and not sluggish.

Flax, chia, and hemp seeds are excellent sources of dietary fiber.

Hemp seeds are the most highly nutritious seeds in the world, packed with fiber, essential fatty acids, vitamins, minerals, and enzymes. They are an excellent source of plant-based protein. I make sure I have a heaping tablespoon in my smoothie every day.

Chia seeds are also an excellent source of essential fatty acids, vitamins, minerals, and fiber. Chia seeds get their name from the ancient Mayan word for *strength*. These tiny seeds are valued for their energy-boosting properties. Chia seeds control your hunger since they absorb ten times their weight in liquid, making them an ideal weight-loss food.

Flaxseeds are one of the oldest fiber crops in the world and contain essential fatty acids, vitamins, minerals, and fiber as well as alpha-linolenic acid and omega-3.

Flaxseeds, hemp seeds, and chia seeds are wonderful additions to oatmeal, smoothies, and salads.

Healthy Fats

You need healthy fats from nature as part of your diet, and eating nuts and seeds helps ensure that your fat intake comes from healthy sources. Walnuts, almonds, pistachios, Brazil nuts, pumpkin, sunflower, chia, hemp, and flaxseeds boost your healthy fat intake because they all contain alpha-linolenic acid, a type of omega-3 fatty acid, as well as protein, vitamins, minerals, and dietary fiber.

All nuts and seeds also contain the anti-nutrient *phytase* and require soaking for better digestion.

Soaking Nuts and Seeds

> Add:
> 1–2 tablespoons of unrefined salt
> 2–4 cups raw organic nuts or seeds to a medium-sized bowl

Cover them with pure water. Allow to stand covered on the counter overnight or for 8 hours. Then drain and rinse nuts or seeds. Spread out nuts or seeds in a single layer on a rack to dehydrate at a low temperature no higher than 150°F. You also can achieve this in your conventional oven on a low temperature of 150°F degrees for 12–24 hours.

Barley

Barley is a member of the grass family and has gained popularity as a cereal grain. Barley was one of the first cultivated grains nearly thirteen thousand years ago and is now grown worldwide. Barely makes a wonderful side dish, or an addition to a hot soup due to its chewy texture and nutty taste.

When the weather is cold, a big pot of soup simmering on the stove warms the house as well as the body. Adding some whole grain barley to the pot will improve your health along with keeping you warm. In addition to barley's robust flavor, it is a good source of manganese, dietary fiber, selenium, copper, vitamin B1, chromium, phosphorus, magnesium, and niacin. Barley is a super powerhouse grain at my table, and I hope you make it one at yours.

In addition to the nutrients mentioned above, barley is loaded with complex carbohydrates, soluble and insoluble fiber, sodium, fatty acids, and amino acids. Barley does contain small amounts of gluten and may be difficult to digest for some individuals.

Rye

Rye is a cereal grain that is a member of the wheat tribe and closely related to the barley family. The health benefits of rye are organic compounds, which include manganese, copper, magnesium, phosphorous, B-complex vitamins, dietary fiber, and phenolic antioxidant compounds.

Rye is often considered a superior grain to wheat in terms of weight-loss efforts. Rye bread has become popular since it is typically denser than bread made with wheat flour. Rye is somewhat unique in its extreme binding properties with water molecules. When eating rye, you feel full quickly, which makes rye great for dieters. The nutrient density in rye grain is a great way to healthfully sustain you.

Sourdough

What exactly is sourdough?

The history of sourdough is as old as leavened bread itself.

Sourdough starter is a natural leaven consisting of fermented dough, typically a mixture of grains and liquid. Humans first started using sourdough about six thousand years ago when we brewed grains into beverages and then later baked them into bread. It took about three different yeasts and five strains of bacteria to form a stable culture. Although the benefits and principles of sourdough remain the same, the yeast and *lactobacillus* bacteria are what make the culture quite stable.

A Note of Caution

Your typical baker's yeast does not have any similarity to real sourdough. Baker's yeast cannot survive the acidity in a sourdough culture, so I don't recommend using commercial baker's yeast in a starter.

Sourdough benefits are similar to the benefits of sprouting and soaking. Sourdough germinates by removing the phytase, making the nutrients come alive and the bread more digestible. When looking for real sourdough bread, search for few simple ingredients, such as organic rye, sea salt, sourdough, spelt, and water. If there is any added yeast, using the word *yeast* in the list of ingredients, then it's not real sourdough bread.

For more instruction on creating your own sourdough starter, I recommend Sarah Pope's article at westonprice.org/sarahpope. Since 2002, Sarah has been an educator and chapter leader of The Weston Price Foundation. The Weston Price Foundation is a nonprofit organization "dedicated to challenging diet dictocrats within conventional nutrition circles with historically and anthropologically accurate nutritional guidelines" (Pope, 2016).

The Fuss About Gluten

As a holistic practitioner, I am amazed at how many people avoid gluten, but don't know or understand what it is.

Gluten is a protein found in grains, particularly wheat, and is the most commonly consumed protein source on planet Earth. Gluten is a mixture of two proteins: *gliadin*, a prolamin, gluten protein and *glutenin*, a glutelin protein. Gluten helps certain grains hold their shape, acting as a glue-like substance holding food together. Gluten nourishes plant embryos during germination, a process by which a plant grows from a seed. Gluten gives baked wheat goods their chewiness and elastic texture.

Gluten is a naturally occurring, digestible protein. When the grain is organically grown and is an ancient form of wheat such as spelt, kamut, and einkorn, gluten is perfectly safe for most individuals. Gluten naturally contains phosphorus, vitamin D, folate, calcium, iron, and the B vitamins, which include riboflavin a.k.a. B12, B6, thiamine, and niacin.

Worried about gluten?

Gluten is *not* the real problem. The real problem is the source of the wheat. The worst thing we can do is consume the modern processed gluten-free foods that are highly inflammatory and disease-forming.

The Problem of Modern Gluten

Einkorn, spelt, and kamut are the original and first-documented wheats. They contain small amounts of gluten. These forms of wheat were well digested by humans for thousands of years. They were properly grown without the use of chemical fertilizers and genetic engineering that created *super gluten*. Super gluten is gluten with a much larger molecular structure caused by genetic engineering. Super gluten is a new species of wheat that is resistant to drought and weather resistant, leaving the wheat less much nutritious than the earlier kinds of wheat.

Genetically engineered wheat is wheat that has been manipulated by its genome, a haploid set of chromosomes in a microorganism of complete DNA, including its own genes using biotechnology. Biotechnology, or *gene splicing*, is the technology by which the DNA of one organism is cut and a gene from an unrelated or foreign organism is inserted, giving the original species the characteristics of the other.

Unlike modern wheat, the wheat in ancient and biblical times was completely tolerable when consumed. It was also properly prepared by soaking, the process that germinates the grain for better assimilation of nutrients. There is absolutely nothing wrong with gluten; it is the source of wheat that is the problem.

Einkorn, kamut, and spelt all have an entirely different genetic makeup than modern wheat. These ancient species are considered more nutritious than modern wheat, with higher levels of protein, essential fatty acids, phosphorous, potassium, pyridoxine, and beta-carotenes.

Modern wheats have been hybridized through years, making them indigestible and inflammatory. *Hybridization* is the process of atomic orbitals fused to create new atomic orbitals. The main goal of hybridization has been to increase yields, fight against plant disease, pests, and weather conditions. I believe that hybridization may very well be an additional part of the equation for the rising number of people with a high intolerance to gluten.

Difficult to Digest

Modern wheat has a totally different molecular structure than ancient wheat. Most modern wheat is a hybrid of many different grains and grasses. There are well over twenty-five thousand species of modern wheat. Ancient wheat was mainly one species and contained fourteen chromosomes, whereas modern wheat has forty-two chromosomes. This genetic alteration changed gluten's molecular structure. This hybrid change in chromosomes makes modern wheat extremely difficult to digest.

The molecular structure of modern wheat is twenty-eight times larger than ancient wheat, making it extremely difficult for the body to break down. Spelt, einkorn, kamut, emmer, and farro are the oldest forms of wheat and successfully tolerated by most. These forms of wheat date back well over ten thousand years and are making a major comeback in today's modern health food industry.

People feel a whole lot better when they remove modern gluten from their diet.

Roundup Ready Wheat

Ninety-five percent of modern wheat has been grown with the use of Roundup, a genetically engineered herbicide. Roundup contains *glyphosate*, which significantly disrupts the functioning of beneficial bacteria in the gut and contributes to damage of the intestinal wall. It is obvious that consumption of modern wheat is responsible for digestive disorders, specifically celiac disease, allergies, autoimmune diseases, infertility, and cancer.

Gluten-containing grains that are not properly prepared and are grown with chemical fertilizers make them highly *in*digestible. Gluten is the culprit behind celiac disease, the result of eating modern wheat. Celiac disease is a condition in which the small intestine becomes hypersensitive to gluten; and therefore, antibodies develop creating celiac, an autoimmune disorder. Celiac disease leads to difficulty digesting foods that contain gluten.

Eventually other serious health conditions may occur including:

- Dermatitis (skin rash)
- Anemia
- Osteoporosis
- Infertility
- Miscarriage
- Epilepsy
- Migraines

- Type 1 diabetes
- Intestinal cancers

When I work with a celiac patient, I first put them on a strict, high-probiotic, anti-inflammatory regimen that excludes all grains and processed foods until the inflammation and antibodies have gone away. Once the body is totally healed, then they can slowly introduce heirloom forms of wheat that are properly germinated.

These patients can safely eat specific sources of einkorn or spelt without any problem. The bottom line is to heal the body through a high-probiotic nutritional program and totally avoid the processed empty calories in modern grains including wheat. Clearly everyone should avoid the wheat of modern civilization whether they have celiac or not.

You can rest easy; gluten is not the issue. It is obviously the source of the wheat that is the issue.

Glyphosate and Gluten Conclusion

Humans exposed to glyphosate become even more vulnerable to the damaging effects of other chemicals and environmental toxins. Glyphosate exposure may occur through the use of Roundup on their weeds or through ingestion of its residues on industrialized food products.

The negative impact of glyphosate exposure is slow and insidious over time—months, even years. Glyphosate has an accumulative effect on the cellular systems of the body. Glyphosate, the primary herbicide in Roundup, is used on most genetically altered crops, including wheat, here in the United States. It is a lethal toxin.

Here is a list of most of the inflammatory diseases glyphosate is responsible for:

- Gastrointestinal disorders
- Obesity
- Diabetes
- Heart disease
- Depression
- Autism
- Infertility
- Multiple sclerosis
- Alzheimer's disease
- Asthma
- Allergies
- Infertility
- Digestive disorders
- Degenerative issues
- Many forms of cancer

Gluten-Free Products

Most gluten-free products on the market today are highly processed and contain genetically altered potato, corn, or soy flour. These products usually contain canola and soy oil, that are both genetically modified crops. This doesn't make them a healthy choice simply because they are absent of gluten. These gluten-free sources are highly inflammatory processed foods which should be avoided.

Perfectly healthy and natural gluten-free foods include:

- Brown rice
- Amaranth
- Buckwheat

- Quinoa
- Millet
- Organic corn

When choosing gluten-free breads, please avoid canola, added sugar, soy, and other ingredients that look like they need to be in a science lab. Be sure to also look for ancient grains, organic products, and preparations such as sprouting or fermenting (as in sourdough).

Beware Whole-Grain Breads

Remember this word of caution on *whole wheat bread* or *whole grain wheat bread*. Commercial whole wheat bread is refined, highly processed, genetically altered and contains a laundry list of disease-forming ingredients that are not fit for human consumption. Consumption of these refined whole wheat breads have been responsible for digestive issues, allergies, skin rashes, autoimmune conditions, and heart disease. Even organic whole grain or whole wheat bread can present similar health problems simply because of the source of wheat, the refining of the wheat, the lack of proper grain preparation, as well as unnecessary, harmful ingredients added for additional flavor and color.

Healthy Bread Products

Beware long lists of ingredients. Instead, search for these words:

- Organic
- Ancient grains
- Sprouted or sourdough
- No added sugars
- Real foods in a short list

Look for ancient, sprouted, and organic flours. Or you can sprout ancient grains yourself.

Let's break down these gluten-free ancient grains for better understanding.

Millet

Millet is a fast-growing plant that is cultivated in warm regions around the world as a cereal crop for human food. Millet is a healthy grain that offers a wide range of nutritional value including folate, magnesium, calcium, phosphorus, and zinc. Millet is an excellent food for people with blood sugar issues since it has a low impact on blood sugar. Millet supports cardiovascular health since it is high in dietary fiber, an aid in combatting heart disease. This butter-colored grain has a mild, nutty flavor, yet tastes similar to corn.

This hearty grain will not only sustain you, but will fully nourish you as a complete meal. It also makes a wonderful side dish to compliment a meal. I like millet as a hot breakfast porridge topped with raw butter or ghee, cinnamon, and any fresh fruit. Millet does not need to be soaked since it has low levels of phytase. However, ultra-sensitive individuals may benefit from soaking the millet before cooking.

Keep in mind that 1 cup of raw millet yields about 3½ cups of cooked millet.

Buckwheat

Don't let the name fool you; buckwheat does not contain any wheat and is naturally gluten free. Buckwheat is not a grain, it's a fruit seed that comes from a plant called beech wheat.

Buckwheat's Latin name is *Fagopyrum esculentum,* which belongs to the polygonaceae family of flowering plants.

Buckwheat is packed with fiber, vitamins, and minerals, including iron, zinc, copper, magnesium calcium, phosphorus, and selenium. Buckwheat consumption has been shown to improve heart health by lowering blood pressure. It is nonallergenic and contains large amounts of disease-fighting antioxidants. This combination makes buckwheat a healthy food source.

Buckwheat has become one of my favorites for its earthy, woody flavor. Buckwheat makes a great side dish or even a hearty main dish with some added grass-fed ground beef and a side of raw sauerkraut. This is one of my husband's most popular Ukrainian dishes, as buckwheat is part of his Ukraine heritage.

Now you can imagine how much buckwheat I have eaten in the last two decades.

Quinoa

Quinoa is actually a seed that is naturally gluten free. It is one of only a few plant foods that are considered a complete protein. While it is a great source of iron, lysine, magnesium, vitamin E, and riboflavin (B2), it contains twice as much fiber as most other grains. I love quinoa for its versatility: eaten as a cold salad, a warm side, or even with a hearty bowl of chicken soup.

Rice

Rice is the seed of the grass species called *Oryxa sativa* (Asian rice) or *Oryxa glaberrima* (African Rice). Rice is also called *swamp grass*, cultivated as a cereal grain. Rice is the most widely consumed staple food in the world, particularly in Asia. Rice is the agricultural commodity with the third-highest worldwide production.

There are many different species of rice. As with all foods, I believe that rice in its original form is the most nutritious. I am a wild-food girl, so my favorite is wild rice. Brown rice and wild rice have not been stripped, bleached, or enriched with synthetic vitamins.

White rice, whether organic or not, is not a wise choice. White rice has been stripped, losing all its bran and most of its fiber. This process makes it a binding, nutrient-less starch, increasing your risk of type 2 diabetes. Brown and wild rice are full of naturally occurring nutrients such as selenium, which reduces the risk for developing common illnesses such as diabetes, cancer, heart disease, and arthritis. The effects of consuming white rice are like that of eating white table sugar.

One cup of brown rice provides 80 percent of your daily manganese requirements. Manganese helps the body synthesize fats. Whole grain rice is another excellent source of dietary fiber. Fiber keeps you regulated and reduces your risk of colon cancer. Fiber attaches to substances that cause cancer, as well as to toxins in the body, eliminating them and keeping them from attaching to the colon wall.

Whole grain rice also contains high levels of antioxidants, which are known to prevent free radical damage that leads to oxidative stress, accelerated aging, heart disease, and cancer.

Now I know what you want to ask me, so here's your answer. These grains still should be soaked, as they do contain phytase. However, these grains do not contain the same levels of this enzyme inhibitor as wheat and oats. Individuals who do not have high sensitivities may consume them without soaking.

My suggestion would be to soak them for better nutrient availability, as I believe that food in its most digestible form is healthiest.

Amaranth

Amaranath is an earthy, nutty-tasting seed comparable to brown rice. It has been used as food for more than eight thousand years. Amaranth is naturally gluten free and an excellent source of protein. It is an ancient Aztec staple food and has essential amino acids, including lysine, an amino acid that most other grains are lacking. Amaranath can be enjoyed as a hot breakfast porridge, as a savory side dish, or as an addition to soup or stews in place of potatoes and noodles.

Pasta Lovers, Let's Talk

Most pasta eaters consume semolina pasta, which makes the pasta belly distend at the dinner table, so your pants need unzipping. This was a common occurrence in my Italian household growing up. If this sounds familiar to you, please read on.

Semolina is coarsely made flour made from durum wheat and is used in making pasta, breakfast cereals, muffins, bagels, breads, and couscous. Semolina does contain gluten in an indigestible form, making it troublesome for people with celiac disease. It causes gas, bloating, and digestive upset in individuals who are gluten intolerant. Remember, semolina is a *modern* form of wheat that has enlarged chromosomes. Digestive distress is caused by the size of semolina's molecular chromosomes in its gluten, which are much larger than the gluten of ancient wheat. Gluten that comes from ancient wheat only contains fourteen chromosomes. Semolina contains forty-two chromosomes, making it an indigestible protein.

Semolina does have some nutritional value, such as B-complex vitamins, especially folate and thiamin. However, semolina is not the best source of these nutrients. Semolina is not an ancient form of wheat. It has been bred many generations out of its origin. This process crossbreeds different strains of wheat, changing the original traits of the plant. Although plant breeding has been practiced for thousands of years, modern plant breeding generates foods with undesirable traits, some of which are hazardous to human health. These undesirable traits of modern plant breeding reduce crop genetic diversity, create vulnerability to crops, and cause repercussions in climate and agricultural practices.

Although the nutrients in semolina sound like a power-packed meal, there are much wiser choices providing these same nutrients. Organic semolina pastas and breads are not much better. Though they may be free of genetic mutations and chemical fertilizers, they still cause the same exact effect on blood sugar.

My suggestions for pasta are pastas made from quinoa, millet, brown rice, spelt, kamut, or most ancient grains discussed in this chapter. The best pasta to consume is sprouted ancient grain pasta. If pasta does not say *sprouted,* then it may be difficult to digest due to the presence of phytase, that antinutrient present in grains mentioned above.

Last but Not Least, Cereal Lovers

What are we pumping American children with today? Highly nutritious meals or inflammatory-disease-forming bowls of poison?

Cereal is one of the biggest health disasters in the modern food industry. Yet boxed cereal is promoted by so-called leading health experts as a healthy choice. Cereal is not only refined, it is extruded at extremely high temperatures, making any possible nutrition more difficult to break down and assimilate. Commercial, boxed cereals are full of sugar as well as artificial colors and flavors, genetically modified ingredients, and chemical fertilizers.

Consuming these forms of wheat creates a storage of energy into fat. It is unfair to blame ancient wheat for the health issues associated with modern wheat.

How did an ancient food staple become a toxic junk food?

Children today are overfed, undernourished, yet starving for proper nutrition. Many children are suffering from hyperactivity, attention deficient disorder, and other brain and neurological disorders due to lack of nutrition and ingestion of chemical compounds found exclusively in boxed cereals. Allergies, digestive disorders, and skin issues are also major complaints.

Now that you've placed your spoon down in sheer terror, let me frighten you just a little bit more. What about *organic* boxed cereal? Well, it's not much better. It goes through the same exact processing as conventional boxed cereal, making its grains difficult to digest. Organic cereals are, however, free from chemical fertilizers and genetic mutations.

We need to go beyond organic. We should make our own cereal with dried organic berries, organic coconut flakes, raw sprouted nuts, sprouted ancient grains, and one of nature's delicious sweeteners, such as raw honey or fresh fruit.

Alternatively, we can look for cereals that have these exact characteristics, which are becoming more readily available online and in health food stores worldwide. This same information also pertains to granola and cereal bars.

By the way, breakfast is not the most important meal of the day. This myth was created by the cereal companies to sell more cereal. Breaking your fast is not a meal. Upon arising, hydration should occur first to allow your pancreas and liver to excrete the necessary enzymes that work as the catalyst that you need to break down your food. Consuming a heavy meal first thing in the morning is **not** what the doctor ordered. Eating too soon after you awaken can create over-worked organs, as well as future health issues.

Cereal Grasses

Cereal grasses are the young green plants that grow to eventually produce cereal grain. These young grasses are the green leaves of wheat, barley, kamut, rye, and oats, which are what I like to call the *infants* of most grains, typically the grains discussed in the beginning of this chapter.

Raw juices in the form of cereal grasses, such as oat grass, wheat grass, and barley grass are some of the most nutrient-rich foods on the planet. Cereal grasses contain large amounts of chlorophyll, which is the *blood* of plants, making it an excellent blood purifier for humans. Cereal grasses are a great way to begin your morning. Breaking your fast with heavy food creates indigestion and doesn't allow your body to fully heal after your fast. Breaking a fast with fresh raw juices is a great way to encourage optimal health. Cereal grasses can be found as green powders to add to juices, water, or smoothies.

One of my morning rituals is sixteen ounces of water with two tablespoons of raw apple cider vinegar and probiotic supplementation. Twenty minutes to about a half an hour later, I have freshly made juice with organic ingredients and added cereal grass powders.

I do not consume solids in the morning until around 11:30. This method of eating will allow your body to rest and heal at the proper times, enhancing healthy digestion that leads to wellness and longevity.

Suggestions for healthy grains can be found in the resource section at the back of this book.

CHAPTER THIRTEEN

Not Too Salty, Not Too Sweet

Salt and sugar consumption are topics of concern for our health, so allow me to give you a thorough description of what makes them bittersweet.

The Difference Between Salt and Sugar

The answer is quite simple; salt is sodium chloride and sugar is sucrose. Keep in mind that the ending -*ose* indicates a form of sugar, but let's break down the differences a bit more thoroughly.

Salt and sugar may appear similar, but they behave differently from one another. Salt is composed of ions that form a crystal through ionic bonding; sugar is composed of molecules bonded together based on positively and negatively charged areas. In salt, the positive and negative areas of water molecules are attracted to ions that are oppositely charged. With sugar, the positive and negative areas of water molecules are attracted to the positive and negative areas on sugar molecules (Chemistry Review, 2016). Sugar and salt atoms bond together differently; and therefore, water interacts and dissolves salt and sugar in distinctive ways.

REFINED AND UNREFINED SALT

Refined Salt

Many people ask me if sea salt is better than refined table salt. Since most salt comes from the sea, the real difference is what happened to it before it arrived at your dinner table. White table salt is bleached, fluorinated, chlorinated, and refined. It's brined in a solution that may include sulfuric acid or chlorine. Then it is heated to a point that removes the necessary minerals and elements beneficial to our bodies.

To extend the shelf life of refined salt, an anti-caking agent, *aluminum silicate*, is added. This chemical is a colorless, odorless crystal that is synthetically produced of silicon, sodium, aluminum, and oxygen. It is also a primary contributor to Alzheimer's disease.

Real, unrefined salt contains naturally occurring iodine, a necessary mineral for healthy thyroid function. Artificial iodine is added to refined salt to prevent thyroid conditions, such as goiters. Unfortunately, this additive is a miniscule amount of .01 percent. This amount is insufficient for the body's iodine needs, as well as being from an artificial source. Bleached, fluorinated, white, refined table salt that you buy in supermarkets or use as a condiment when you dine out has absolutely no resemblance to real, unrefined sea salt.

When this highly poisonous refined salt is absorbed by the body, it eventually causes water retention. Your hands and legs swell, and your blood pressure may spike. Refined salt consumption over time causes high blood pressure, as well as placing a heavy burden on your kidneys. Original sea salt is also treated with lime or caustic soda to remove the magnesium, an extremely critical mineral for the heart, brain, and central nervous system. Most of the other valuable minerals in the original sea salt are also lost or extracted in the refining process.

Most people on a Standard American Diet (SAD) crave salt because their bodies are craving the other trace minerals once present in sea salt before the refining process. The loss of these necessary minerals has led to excessive food addictions – that are partly responsible for today's obesity epidemic.

Eliminating processed foods is the best way to cut down on your refined salt intake since these *foods* are heavily laden with processed salt.

> *You are the salt of the earth, but if salt has lost its taste, how shall its saltiness be restored? It is no longer good for anything except to be thrown out and trampled under people's feet.*
>
> – Matthew 5:13 ESV

Unrefined Salt

Unrefined salt is real sea salt that's unbleached and unprocessed. This salt contains trace minerals that occur naturally, including iodine. It is never exposed to fluoride, synthetic processing, or bleaching agents.

Unrefined salt is much more than just sodium and chloride; it is a whole food that is recognized and used by the body. Unrefined salt provides up to ninety-two necessary minerals that balance all bodily systems, including the immune, glandular, the brain, and nervous systems.

I encourage you to switch to real, unrefined salt in your diet, if you have not already. Salt has had a bad rap for a few decades now. However, our bodies are starving for the benefits that are locked into real salt. Refined salt causes high blood pressure.

But did you know that insufficient amounts of real, unrefined salt also elevate blood pressure?

Let's take a close look at all the amazing benefits of real, unrefined salt.

Real salt is a strong, natural antihistamine that is beneficial for those suffering from allergies. It prevents muscle cramps. The minerals in real salt are natural electrolytes that keep the body in balance while giving your body a positive electrical charge that prevents and reverses dehydration.

The naturally occurring minerals in unrefined salt help to prevent excess saliva production. Saliva that is flowing out of the mouth during sleep may be an indication of a salt mineral deficiency. Real salt makes bones and teeth strong by rebuilding bone mineral density and osteoblast cells. The minerals found in real salt are the same minerals that are necessary for healthy bones. Perhaps this explains why those eating refined salt suffer from of osteoporosis.

Real unrefined salt:

- Is a natural hypnotic
- Regulates heartbeat
- Induces sleep
- Alkalizes the blood
- Prevents gout
- Prevents spider veins
- Maintains a healthy libido
- Balances blood pressure
- Balances blood glucose levels

Lastly, unrefined salt is needed to clear the lungs of mucus, sticky phlegm, catarrh, and congestion particularly in those suffering from colds, flus, asthma, and cystic fibrosis.

Have I encouraged you enough to start consuming this fabulous salt?

There are several different types of unrefined salt that contain necessary trace minerals due to the place of its origin. These include Celtic sea salt, pink Himalayan salt, Hawaiian salt, and Icelandic flake salt. I use and highly recommend these salts.

Now keep in mind that these unrefined salts are equal in quality due to their superior mineral content and their lack of refining and processing. Each salt, though, has a slight difference in flavor. The choice is based on your personal taste preference.

Using Real Salt

Use real salt as you would normally use refined salt. However, real salt is stronger in taste since the flavor, minerals, and nutrients have not been altered or stripped away—so less is more.

Take a quick look below at my favorite salts and remember these salts each have the medicinal benefits mentioned above.

Celtic Sea Salt

Celtic sea salt is a grey-colored natural, unrefined salt that provides an important source of sodium chloride, a naturally occurring mineral critical for good health. Celtic Sea Salt is abundant in potassium, magnesium, selenium, and other important trace minerals. Celtic sea salt is available in fine and coarse ground.

Hawaiian Black Lava or Red Alaea Sea Salt

Hawaiian salts—whether red, black, or pinkish brown—are unrefined sea salts that contain numerous amounts of critical trace minerals. Their pink and brownish colors come from particles of volcanic red clay. Black Lava Sea Salt derives its color from activated coconut shell charcoal. Hawaiian salt comes in pyramid-shape flakes, ranging from fine to coarse grain.

Himalayan Sea Salt

Himalayan is the purest form of sea salt since it is harvested from ancient sea beds that have been protected from modern pollution. Himalayan pink salt receives its color from iron oxide and the presence of eighty-four trace minerals. Himalayan Sea Salt offers minerals similar to the ones listed above, making it another wonderful source of salt to add to your condiment list. Even though pink salt crystals come from mountains, they are still considered sea salt since all salt comes from a salted body of water.

Icelandic Flake Sea Salt

Icelandic flake salt is crunchy, white, and flakey. This salt is mineral-rich and is the only salt produced from the geothermal energy of hot springs in northeast Iceland. Icelandic flake salt contains the highest mineral content of natural salts, ranking it a top sea salt to add to your cooking, salads, and water for a quick mineral boost.

How Much Salt

Understand that salt is a condiment and should be used in small quantities; you don't need more salt simply because you are excited about the benefits. Real unrefined salt is so mineral rich—remember that less is more. The average person needs approximately ten to twelve pinches, or about three-quarters of a teaspoon, daily. These small portions should be added sporadically on food throughout the day and in water for a quick mineral boost.

An additional amount may be needed after a sweaty workout or in the summer months when you've perspired heavily. The perfect ratio of salt to water—an eighth of teaspoon to sixteen ounces of water—is critical for the mineral benefit, as well as hydration. Be sure to consume about sixty-four ounces of pure water daily.

A Great Headache Remedy

Ten ounces of room-temperature water with ⅛ of any of these real salts can fix a mineral deficiency that leads to a headache. Drinking this mixture twice can ward off a headache without the use of a toxic painkiller.

You May Be Sweet Enough

Now that you are an expert on salt, let's dive right into all the different types of sweeteners. It shouldn't surprise you that our human species has an innate sweet tooth. Although not everyone adores sweets, I would say that most of us do. Let's explore why some of us are sweet enough, and why some of us may not be.

In my opinion, sugar is one of the most dangerous ingredients on the food market. It's addictive and added to almost every processed food. Sugar has the potential to make you depressed, sick, and overweight. Cancer cells feed on sugar. Glucose is an ingredient of the liquid pumped into a cancer patient undergoing a PET scan with contrast because the glucose will find the cancer.

Sugar consumption has doubled in the last thirty years due to the increase of processed and fast food products. Most Americans are now consuming about 150 pounds of sugar every year. Since the overconsumption of this addictive, drug-like, white powder began, the health of this nation has declined. Everything from heart disease, digestive disorders, diabetes, eye problems, thyroid issues, and cancer is on the rise.

What exactly is sugar?

Sugar is a sweet-tasting short-chain, soluble carbohydrate found naturally in most plants, also known as fructose, glucose, or sucrose. A natural substance, sugar is becoming a poison due to its processing and overconsumption.

THE NOT-SO-SWEET SWEETENERS

White Table Sugar

Let's begin with the sweetener that you are most familiar with: simple, white table sugar. White table sugar is refined, bleached, and chlorinated, much like refined salt. Most white sugar today comes from genetically engineered sugar beets, making this white powder an addictive drug. Genetically modified sugar beets are a gene technology crafted by Monsanto, the corporate giant genetically modifying our food supply.

Be aware that excess amounts of sugar cause white blood cells to shut down their ability to ward off disease up to six hours after consumption. When a patient finally realizes that sugar inhibits immune function, it usually hits home.

In the words of the American Anti-Cancer Institute, when we consume sugar, we are simultaneously shutting off our first line of defense against cancer (Axe, 2015). In my opinion, adding sugar to our diet seems even more like suicide.

High Fructose Corn Syrup (HFCS)

High fructose corn syrup is a sweetener made from corn syrup processed to convert glucose into fructose. HFCS is cheaper and sweeter than sugar due to government farm bill corn subsidies, but it costs consumers their health. HFCS boosts your risk of diabetes, high blood pressure, heart disease, and cancer. High fructose corn syrup may also contribute to a fatty liver and liver disease. Regular consumption of foods containing HFCS puts you at an increased risked of developing neuro-degenerative diseases, which include dementia and Alzheimer's disease.

HFCS consists of fructose and glucose in an unbalanced ratio of 55:45, which is why the body has difficulty breaking down this sweetener. The body's digestive enzymes must break down sucrose into glucose and fructose, and then it is absorbed into the body.

High fructose corn syrup is found in almost every processed food on the market:

- Salad dressings
- Juice
- Dairy products
- Frozen dinners

- Boxed cereals
- Cookies
- Yogurt
- Breads
- Baked goods
- Candy
- *Health* bars

HFCS is certainly not the ideal sweetener.

Agave Nectar

Agave nectar is produced in Mexico from the agave tequila plant. Agave is approximately one-and-a-half times sweeter than regular table sugar and contains sixty calories per tablespoon. A tablespoon of regular sugar contains sixteen calories per tablespoon. Agave nectar has become popular in the health-conscious community. Many believe—or should I say have been deceived into thinking—that agave is a wise choice for a sweetener due to its low glycemic index. It has a low, immediate impact on blood glucose levels. However, agave nectar is *worse* than high fructose corn syrup. Just because agave nectar sits on the shelves in a health food store doesn't mean it's healthy.

Most commercial agave nectar is processed using caustic acids and filtration chemicals classified as:

- Activated charcoal
- Inulin enzymes
- Claimex
- Aulfuric
- Hydrofluoric acid

Agave nectar is a laboratory processed, condensed, fructose syrup ranking 75–97 percent higher in fructose than HFCS.

Fructose is a naturally occurring sugar in fruit, giving fruit its sweetness. Your body is designed to handle this type of sugar in small amounts. Your body metabolizes the high levels of fructose in agave the same way it metabolizes chronic alcohol consumption. The extremely high amounts of fructose in agave nectar play havoc on the liver, causing a fatty liver and nonalcoholic liver disease.

Whether agave is organic or not, it still has the potential to cause serious health issues due to its high fructose content. Like HFCS, agave nectar tricks your body into gaining weight by impairing your body`s metabolism and increasing your appetite control systems.

In addition, agave nectar consumption can cause:

- Insulin resistance
- Type 2 diabetes
- Adrenal fatigue
- Depleted metabolism
- Cancer

I would suggest avoiding agave nectar as your choice of sweetener.

ARTIFICIAL SWEETENERS

Aspartame

In my days of yo-yo dieting, aspartame was a common ingredient on my shopping list. I suffered many health challenges due to this not-so-sweet sweetener.

Aspartame is a highly sweet substance used as an artificial sweetener, mainly in low-calorie products.

These products include:

- Diet soda
- Sugar-free pudding
- Sugar-free gelatin
- Fruit spreads
- Reduced-calorie fruit juice
- Chewable vitamins
- Sugar-free cough drops
- Light yogurt
- Sugarless candy and gum
- Diet or reduced-fat baked goods

Aspartame is the most dangerous additive on the market today.

This artificially sweet poison is most often labeled on a product as *phenylalanine* and is a derivative of aspartic acid and phenylalanine. Aspartame is sold under the brand names NutraSweet and Equal.

The Making of Aspartame

Aspartame is made from feces of genetically engineered *E. coli* bacteria, that are cultivated in tanks and fed so they can excrete the proteins that contain phenylalanine and aspartic acid.

Who *dreams* up these things?

Side effects of aspartame consumption may include:

- Headaches
- Skin issues
- Dizziness
- Digestive symptoms
- Anxiety attacks
- Weight gain

- Nausea
- Numbness
- Blurred vision
- Mood changers
- More serious health issues associated with aspartame include:
- Breathing difficulties
- Birth defects
- Diabetes
- Attention deficit disorder
- Seizure disorder
- Chronic fatigue syndrome
- Parkinson disease
- Alzheimer's disease
- Lupus
- Brain lesions
- Severe memory loss
- Cancer
- ALS (amyotrophic lateral sclerosis)
- Dementia
- Brain lesions
- Lymphoma
- Epilepsy
- Multiple sclerosis

Researchers of the Columbia University and at the University of Miami discovered that consuming one diet soda per day for up to ten years increased risk of heart disease and stroke (Gardener, 2012).

How Aspartame Causes Damage

Excitotoxins are substances that stimulate taste receptors on the tongue, exciting or stimulating neural cells to death. *Excitotoxicity* is the pathological process by which nerve cells are damaged or killed. The neural cell damage caused by excessive amounts of aspartate and the neurotransmitter glutamate is why these substances are referred to as *excitotoxins*. Both substances are present in aspartame.

In addition, these taste receptors, along with pathologically high levels of glutamate, can cause excitotoxicity by allowing high levels of calcium to enter cells. Aspartame consumption produces excessive amounts of free radicals, causing cellular death.

This highly dangerous, unnatural process of aspartame certainly makes this sweetener an *unwise* choice.

For additional research on this issue, I highly suggest the book, *Excitotoxins: The Taste that Kills*, by Russell L. Blaylock, MD, a retired neurosurgeon and health pioneer (Blaylock, 1994).

Splenda

We have been brainwashed to believe that Splenda is a form of sugar and somehow safer than other artificial sweeteners on the market. Truthfully, Splenda is an artificial, chlorinated sweetener responsible for many health issues.

Splenda consumption increases blood glucose levels, despite being marketed as a safe alternative for diabetics. Splenda accumulates in the body since the body does not know how to process it. It is stored in fat tissue or even in the brain, possibly contributing to Alzheimer`s and Parkinson`s diseases.

Splenda consumption has also contributed to:

- Migraines
- Dizziness
- Intestinal cramping
- Rashes
- Acne
- Headaches
- Bloating
- Chest pain
- Tinnitus
- Gum bleeding
- Tooth decay

Consequently, Splenda alters hormones and depletes metabolism, which promotes weight gain.

Natural News (naturalnews.com) explains why Splenda might taste like sugar, but is a pesticide poison in disguise:

> Splenda contains a lethal substance called organochlorine pesticide compound, similar to (DDT) a synthetic, organic compound used as an insecticide, and (PCBs) a polychlorinated biphenyls, and other harmful substances that are not fit for human consumption. When heated alongside other foods, Splenda can degrade into other toxic compounds known as persistent organic pollutants, or POPs. Splenda undergoes a thermal degradation process that results in the formation of cancer-causing dioxin and dioxin-like compounds. During the process of this breakdown, certain chlorine compounds are released that create geno-toxic, carcinogenic, and tumorigenic characteristics.

Splenda is also partially metabolized upon ingestion, contrary to what McNeil Nutritionals, LLC, its manufacturer claims. A 2013 study published in the *Journal of Toxicology and Environmental Health* found that while some Splenda passes through the body undigested, some is also absorbed during digestion. Although early studies asserted that sucralose passes through the GIT (gastrointestinal tract) unchanged, subsequent analysis suggested that some of the ingested sweetener is metabolized in the GIT, as indicated by multiple peaks found in thin-layer radio chromatographic profiles of methanolic fecal extracts after oral sucralose administration, explains the study, which observed noticeable damage from sucralose ingestion on beneficial gut bacteria (Huff, 2014).

This zero-calorie sweetener is an extremely poor choice and should be on your dangerous sweetener check *off* list.

Raw Sugar, a.k.a. Turbinado Sugar

There are only four kinds of sugar: white, light brown, dark brown, and raw. Sugars go under the names: pure sugarcane, turbinado sugar, and brand names Sugar in the Raw and Sucanat. All forms of nonwhite sugars are made from a base of white sugar with added molasses, making them a tiny bit better tasting than white sugar, but still just as unhealthy as the pure white version.

These so-called healthier alternatives to white sugar all contain 99.96 percent sucrose, which is potentially harmful when frequently consumed.

I am frequently asked about raw sugar. I am also asked of if using brown sugar instead of white sugar is a healthier option.

Sugar in the Raw is a brand name that is deceiving, and it's found in every coffee shop around the globe. Coffee drinkers add this sweetener as an alternative to regular table sugar, believing they have made a healthier choice. *Turbinado* is another name for raw sugar. It comes from the process used to make it. Turbinado is made by crushing the freshly-cut sugarcane, evaporating and crystallizing it, and then spinning it in a turbine to remove most of the molasses — which gives its light brown color. Other than color, the residual molasses gives turbinado sugar its flavor and texture.

There's good news and bad news about brown sugars. The good news is there are nutrients present, such as B vitamins, calcium, iron, and potassium in minimal amounts. White sugar goes through a refining process, and the molasses is totally removed from the sugarcane crystals. Bleaching agents and chlorine are also used in the refining process of white sugar. Light and dark brown sugars are made by adding different amounts of the molasses back into refined sugar to give it a brownish color and flavor. Molasses is about 60 percent sugar, but contains small amounts of trace minerals. However, the bad news is that turbinado sugar has the same effects on blood glucose levels as does white sugar.

Sugar in the Raw isn't actually raw or unrefined. Turbinado sugar is what's *left over* after raw sugarcane juice has been refined and stripped of its natural molasses and impurities, as well as its vitamins and minerals, making the product less nutritious and more difficult to digest.

Blackstrap Molasses

Blackstrap Molasses is a sweet, robust-tasting, thick liquid that results from processing sugar cane into white table sugar. It is wonderful in baking or added to your favorite hot beverage as a nourishing tonic.

This dark syrup is loaded with minerals and nutrients and is known for its high iron content, making it an excellent source of sweetener for those suffering from iron deficiency. Molasses also works as a gentle laxative by drawing water to the stool for an easier smooth move.

Please be aware that all forms of sugar:

- Rob the body of B vitamins
- Disrupt calcium metabolism
- Create mineral deficiencies
- Increase risks of heart disease
- Increase risk of cancer
- Impair cognition
- Over-activate brain receptors that hinder cravings and mood swings

All processed sugar is bad for you.

These processed sugars may be slightly less unhealthy than regular, white table sugar, but the chemical structure is exactly the same. Your body won't recognize any difference. No matter which brown sugar you choose—Sugar in the Raw, Sucanat, organic cane sugar—the effect equals regular table sugar. When consuming these sugars, the molecules break down into glucose and fructose in the digestive tract and will all have the same harmful effects on your pancreas and your blood glucose levels. In addition, they slow your metabolism, create fat storage, add unwanted weight, and elevate cholesterol levels.

Whether sugar is raw or not makes no difference to your pancreas. Over-consumption of any sugar creates a higher risk of diabetes, heart disease, and cancer.

Evaporated Cane Juice

I am going to shock you again. Evaporated cane juice is a deceiving marketing strategy to make us think it's healthy. Please don't be fooled by the name; it's a misleading name for plain old sugar.

If you see *evaporated* and *juice* on the ingredient label, it's not a healthier choice. When the sweetener reaches your pancreas and liver, your body won't recognize any difference between *evaporated juice* and plain old sugar, high fructose corn syrup, turbinado, or raw sugar. You're dealing with the same exact side effects as listed above and with similar processing.

Food for Thought

Organically grown sugar is still sugar, so whether it is raw or organic doesn't make any difference. All sugars have a high glycemic load, which creates a rapid delivery into your bloodstream, resulting in the possibility of many side effects. These effects, listed above, are not erased simply because a sugar is organic.

BETTER SWEETENERS

Coconut Sugar

Coconut sugar is the boiled and dehydrated sap of the coconut palm, which is dehydrated and made into sugar. Coconut sugar, also known as coconut palm sugar, has a much lower glycemic index than the above sugars. It may be more expensive and a better sweetener than common table sugar, but still has the same number of carbohydrates and calories.

The Benefits of Coconut Sugar

Coconut sugar offers several nutrients and minerals that are found in the palm, whereas regular table sugar is void of these nutrients.

The nutrients found in coconut sugar in trace amounts include:

- Vitamin C
- Potassium
- Phosphorous
- Magnesium
- Calcium
- Zinc
- Iron
- Copper

Coconut sugar also provides small amounts of phytonutrients, such as polyphenols, flavonoids, inositol, and some antioxidants. The glycemic index of coconut sugar is much lower than the sugars discussed above.

Coconut sugar ranks 35 on the glycemic index while regular table sugar ranks between 60–75. Sugars that are high on the glycemic index cause your blood sugar to spike, leading to a sugar rush followed by a crash. This rush is known as a sugar high and it is followed by a rapid drop. Fast spikes in blood sugar can also cause your insulin levels to elevate in a short time, and this creates problems for diabetics or anyone with sugar sensitivity. Although it is lower on the GI scale, coconut sugar is still sugar and should be consumed in small quantities, especially by sugar-sensitive individuals.

Coconut sugar contains 45 percent fructose, making it a better option than some other sweeteners. However, when your liver breaks down fructose, one of the results is triglyceride, a form of fat. To be healthy, limit your amounts of fructose to what you receive from fresh fruit.

Coconut sugar tastes great and is wonderful in baking, sweetening your coffee and tea, and added to hot and cold cereals.

Coconut Nectar

Raw coconut nectar, or *coconut palm nectar,* is a low glycemic sweetener that comes from the sweet sap of the thick flowering stems of the coconut tree flower blossoms. This sap is evaporated at low temperatures, producing a raw, high enzymatic, nutrient-rich pourable syrup that is wonderful on top of pancakes, waffles, and your favorite dessert.

Low glycemic sweeteners are better choices for most people, but they are especially good for diabetics and those wanting to lose excess body weight. They don't cause blood sugar spikes that may lead to addictive eating behaviors and cravings.

The health benefits of coconut nectar include a rich source of nutrients, vitamins, minerals, and beneficial living enzymes. This sweetener is unrefined and is not chemically treated or processed. This wonderful nectar contains no additives or preservatives. Last, but not least, it tastes amazing.

Coconut nectar is one of my favorite sweeteners.

Maple Syrup

Maple syrup is another favorite sweetener of mine. I love its rich taste on top of pancakes and added to oatmeal. Maple syrup is collected by drilling a hole in, or *tapping,* a maple tree and gathering the crystal-clear sap. The liquid is boiled until most of the water content evaporates or is reduced, creating a thick sugary syrup that is then filtered to remove its impurities. It takes forty gallons of sap to make one gallon of syrup.

Maple syrup is gathered in the early spring, when the change from cool night temperatures to the heat of the sun during the day forces the trees' sap up into the branches and wakes the tree from its winter dormancy. The seasonal flow of the sap is what makes it possible to collect it. Maple syrup is made mostly from the sugar maple, red maple, or black maple, because they have a higher sugar content.

Antioxidants, Vitamins, and Minerals

Maple syrup carries a high nutrition composition, including vitamins, minerals, and anti-inflammatory polyphenols. In small quantities, maple syrup can be part of a healthy diet, reducing your risk of arthritis, digestive issues, heart disease, and cancer. Maple syrup's high antioxidant profile reduces oxidative stress in the body, the main culprit in the depression of the immune system. The antioxidants in maple syrup can protect cells from DNA damage and mutation.

The addition of maple syrup alone won't likely result in the reduction of certain diseases, but will instead contribute to an overall healthy diet.

Maple syrup contains calcium, iron, zinc, phosphorus, sodium, and potassium — all beneficial minerals for a healthy heart and brain. Vitamins in maple syrup include thiamin, niacin, B6, and riboflavin—promoting a healthy metabolism and stress reduction.

Low Glycemic Load

Maple syrup is delicious, and it has a low glycemic index. Using pure maple syrup in place of other sweeteners will do your body good. A glycemic index of 55 or below is considered *low glycemic* and maple syrup has a glycemic index of 54, very good for a sweetener.

Sources

After learning about the amazing benefits of this fabulous sweetener, it is important to find the right source. You must choose pure maple syrup to get these benefits. Be aware of deceiving marketing labels, such as *breakfast* or *pancake* syrups. Also avoid labels that read *light* syrup and *diet* syrup. These common syrups contain absolutely no maple syrup and are made from high-fructose corn syrup, artificial maple flavoring, and caramel coloring. Caramel coloring is a known carcinogen and is also found in breads, prepackaged foods, cakes, cookies, and frozen dinners.

These maple syrup impostors taste artificial and can cause a laundry list of health issues. Keep in mind that pure maple syrup is made from the sap of a maple tree and can never be duplicated using these artificial methods. Aunt Jemima had it all wrong. Be sure to purchase pure maple syrup that is organic, remembering to choose food free of chemical fertilizers and genetic mutations.

There are a variety of grades of maple syrup, ranging from light in color and flavor to dark and robust (my favorite). The lighter grades are used in baking so the maple flavor doesn't overpower the final product. Darker grades are more flavorful, almost nearing molasses. The lighter grades are harvested earlier in the season, usually early February, and the darker ones later. All grades have similar nutritional benefits, so let your taste buds be your guide.

Vermont Fancy

The first syrup produced in the beginning of the maple season is syrup that is graded Vermont Fancy. This syrup is characterized as golden in color, has a delicate, mild flavor, and a hint of vanilla that comes from the vanillin that is naturally present in maple sap. Vermont produces 8 percent of the world's maple syrup, employing strict grading standards that are more comprehensive in classification. Fancy-grade syrup is best drizzled over your favorite desserts. Vermont Fancy is equal in nutrition quality and thickness to other grades; it's a personal taste preference.

As I type this chapter, I can almost taste the sweet, aromatic richness of maple syrup. I bet you can, too. Please take a break and satisfy your taste buds with my coconut banana nut pancakes. Drizzle them with pure, organic maple syrup as your desire.

By the way, whether its morning, afternoon, or dinnertime, pancakes are wonderful for any meal.

Tonijean's Coco Banana Nut Pancake Recipe

Ingredients
  6 pasture-raised eggs
  3 ripe, organic bananas
  2 tablespoons of coconut flour
  1 tablespoon of pure vanilla extract
  ½ cup raw, organic chopped walnuts (optional)
  ½ teaspoon Celtic or pink salt
  1 teaspoon. organic Ceylon cinnamon

In a medium bowl, beat eggs. Add salt, vanilla, nuts, cinnamon, and coconut flour. Mix well.

In a separate bowl, mash bananas well and add to the egg mixture. Mix well with an electric hand mixer on low speed. Heat a stainless or cast iron skillet over medium heat. Add organic butter or unrefined, organic coconut oil, enough to cover pan. Add 2–3 tablespoons of mixture for each pancake and cook 2 minutes on each side or until lightly golden brown. Top with butter or ghee, and pure, organic maple syrup of your choice and a sprinkle of cinnamon.

All sugar sources, including maple syrup, should be used in small quantities and with caution for those having sugar sensitivity.

Raw Honey

Raw honey is one of my top choices of sweeteners, but there are shocking differences between raw honey and the processed honey found on your grocery store's shelves. Honey is a sweet, sticky, yellowish-brown fluid made by bees from flower nectar. Yes, bees are most definitely involved, unlike commercial honey that is nothing but high fructose corn syrup and caramel color. That extremely unhealthy liquid is then pasteurized and presented as honey.

Breaking It Down

Raw honey is a superfood with high antioxidant properties, bioactive components known as bee pollen, and *propolis*. Real honey contains up to eighty different substances important to human nutrition.

Besides glucose and fructose, honey contains:

- The B-complex vitamins
- Vitamins A, C, D, E, and K
- Magnesium
- Sulfur
- Phosphorus
- Iron
- Calcium
- Chlorine
- Potassium
- Iodine
- Sodium
- Copper
- Manganese

The live enzymatic content of real honey is one of the highest of all foods. Real honey also contains antimicrobial, antifungal, antiviral, and antibacterial properties. This may be why honey is used to combat that dry cough or fight the flu.

A teaspoon a day will keep the doctor away.

The Difference

Most processed honey today has been high-heat processed or pasteurized and then filtered, robbing it of its nutritional value and resulting in a product no more valuable than high fructose corn syrup or any other processed sugar product. Processed honey is nothing but liquid poison and should be completely avoided.

Real honey is an instant energy-building food that has no comparison to commercial honey. Real honey contains all the essential minerals necessary for health, the B complex amino acids, enzymes, anti-allergens, and other vital factors. Real honey is practically free of bad bacteria and is considered a natural preservative since it never spoils. Honey has a shelf life of thousands of years.

> *My son, eat honey, for it is good, yes, the honey from the comb is sweet to your taste.*
> —Proverbs 24:13 NAS

Honey History

Real honey has been noted as one of nature's most perfect foods since the beginning of time. Honey was used in ancient and biblical times both as a food and medicine. *Apiculture,* the science of producing honey, originated over three thousand years ago in Northern Israel, around 700 BCE.

For many centuries, honey was regarded as sacred due to its rarity and was used in religious ceremonies to pay tributes to gods. The Bible refers to Israel as the land of milk and honey (Deuteronomy 26:9). According to the Israelites, *milk and honey* is a metaphor for all good things or God's blessings. In history, its use in cooking was reserved for the wealthy since it was so costly that only the rich could afford it.

Honey was successfully used as medicine in ancient times and has made a major comeback today for those same medicinal purposes. Honey must be both raw and unfiltered for maximum effectiveness and health benefits. These life-giving ingredients may be due to the presence of bee pollen and propolis.

> *And you gave them this land, which you swore to their fathers to give them, a land flowing with milk and honey.*
> —Jeremiah 32:22 ESV

Bee Pollen

Bee pollen is a superfood compound—a powerful medicine containing all the vital nutrients required by the human body. Raw honey is a medicinal source of proteins, vitamins, minerals, beneficial fatty acids, carotenoids, and bioflavonoids. These compounds contain antimicrobial, antiviral, antibacterial, and antifungal properties, which are all beneficial in the prevention of infectious diseases and the promotion of overall health.

Propolis

Propolis is the resinous substance bees collect from tree buds. The bees use it to fill cracks and to seal their honeycombs. Propolis was used successfully in ancient times for abscesses and healing wounds. It has antimicrobial, antibacterial, antifungal, and antiviral qualities, as well as anti-inflammatory and antioxidant properties. This substance combines with other nutrients to make raw honey a highly nutritious powerhouse food.

The Glycemic Index

Honey has a healthy glycemic index, meaning that it is slowly absorbed into the bloodstream. It is easy to digest and assimilate. The glycemic index of honey is about 58–65, slightly higher than maple syrup.

Local Doesn't Guarantee Raw or Organic

Local honey isn't necessarily the best. It might be pasteurized. This process alters all the nutritional properties, making this honey an unhealthy sweetener. Ask your local farmers how their honey is processed to ensure that their honey is raw. Also ask if the honey is organic, remembering the importance of food being free of chemical fertilizers and genetic mutations. Looking for honey that is both raw and organic will guarantee you of all its medicinal benefits.

Raw Honey and Allergies

Real, raw, organic honey is full of antiallergenic substances, such as propolis and bee pollen in addition to its abundance of vitamins, minerals, and enzymes. These components play a critical role in the reduction of allergies by exposing the body to miniscule amounts of pollen over time. Keep in mind that as soon as honey is pasteurized, all these vital nutrients are destroyed.

Honey's Not-Sweet Future

It saddens me that scientific reports show real honey may be on the decline due to the destruction of our planet. Everything from chemical fertilizers, genetic engineering, toxic waste spills, oil spills, and other chemical loads, such as electromagnetic radiation pollution, are causing the decline of bees. Honeybees play a critical role in the pollination of most of our plant food crops and without them, we are in serious trouble. The ecological crisis of a declining bee population poses a major threat to worldwide agriculture.

Sources

There are more than three hundred types of honey in the United States alone, each with a unique flavor and color depending on the blossoming flowers and trees visited by bees.

If honey is both raw and organic, then your choice of flavor and color is based on your taste buds.

Other characteristics to look for when purchasing honey:

- Raw
- Organic
- Unfiltered
- Unheated
- Unadulterated
- Unpasteurized
- Local

Honey will crystalize over time, but can be returned to its flowing state by placing it inside a container in a gently heating pan of water.

Pure Green Leaf Stevia

Stevia is an actual sweet leaf and not considered a sugar, yet is forty times sweeter than sugar. Stevia is the only sweetener that is not harmful in any way and also has health benefits. It has no calories, and is 100 percent natural, but you must choose the right one. This green leafy plant is a native to South America. Stevia has been used for medicinal purposes for many centuries. This plant has been bred for its intense, sweet flavor.

Stevia provides the following health benefits:

- Controls and lowers blood pressure
- Lowers blood sugar
- Reduces dandruff and acne
- Protects teeth and gums
- Aids in weight loss
- Aids wound healing
- Helps digestion
- Reduces fine lines and wrinkles

Low Glycemic

Stevia is a non-nutritive sweetener that does not affect blood glucose levels at all. Stevia has a glycemic index score of 0, which means that eating stevia will not raise your blood sugar.

Stevia is a green, leafy herbal plant and there are approximately two hundred species of stevia that grow in South America. What makes stevia leaves sweet are two *glycosides*—*stevioside* and *rebaudioside*. Stevioside is sweet, but also has a bitter aftertaste. I hear complaints about that aftertaste when using stevia. Rebaudioside is better tasting, sweeter, and less bitter.

Less-processed stevia products contain both sweeteners, as the whole stevia leaf is present. Pure stevia contains stevioside as well as rebaudioside. However, you must be aware that refined stevia sweeteners don't resemble the whole stevia plant. Certain brands of stevia are highly processed with added chemicals, making these types of stevia an unhealthy choice.

These include most highly processed forms of stevia, like Truvia, which only contains the rebaudioside, the sweetest part of the stevia leaf. In addition, these highly refined stevia extracts may cause side effects, such as nausea, bloating, or a feeling of an uncomfortable fullness.

Be aware of *maltodextrin* in your stevia. It is derived from plants and used as a food additive or a non-caking agent. The form of maltodextrin used in some stevia products is from genetically modified corn, making it extremely unhealthy.

Liquids, Powders, and Extracts

Whether you choose to purchase extracts, liquid, or powder, here are the sweet leaf conversion amounts, which you may find very helpful.

> 1 tablespoon of powdered stevia = ½ cup regular sugar
> 10 packets of stevia = 1 tablespoon of powdered stevia
> 1 teaspoon of liquid stevia = 1 tablespoon powdered stevia
> 5 droppers of liquid stevia = 1 teaspoon stevia powder
> ¼ teaspoon stevia extract = 2 tablespoons of powdered stevia powder
> ½ teaspoon stevia liquid extract = 2 cups regular sugar

Whether you choose powder, extract, or liquid, you must look for the words *pure green leaf.* These words reflect minimal processing, as well as the highest quality standard of your stevia, to assure you of the nutritional benefits.

Xylitol

Xylitol is a naturally occurring sugar alcohol found in most plant material, including many fruits and vegetables. It is extracted from birch wood to make medicine. Xylitol is used as a sugar replacement in chewing gums, mints, and other candies labeled *sugar-free*. However, it may not be healthy in larger amounts, because the body cannot digest these sugar alcohols properly.

The nonmetabolized portion of sugar alcohol ferments and creates a favorable environment for harmful bacteria. Candida and yeast overgrowth may occur and many people will also experience constipation, gas, bloating, and diarrhea. However, some experts claim that xylitol has powerful benefits for dental health and prevention of tooth decay.

Some sources of xylitol may be under these names: Erythritol, Isomalt, Lactitol, Maltito, Mannitol, and Sorbitol.

My opinion on xylitol is that it should only be used in extremely small quantities, if at all.

Dates and Date Sugar

Date sugar is a wholesome alternative sweetener made from premium quality Deglet Noor dates. The flavor is lightly sweet with a delicious butterscotch essence. Date sugarcane is used in many baking recipes as a one-to-one replacement for white sugar or brown sugar.

This form of sugar comes from dehydrated dates that have been ground into a coarse powder. Date sugar is not low glycemic, even though it is only processed minimally. People with sugar sensitivities should be cautious in its use. Also, dates have a higher fructose ratio and overconsumption of fructose is linked to liver problems and weight gain.

The minimal raw processing of dates allows natural fiber, tannins, flavonoids, vitamins, and minerals to be retained. Keep in mind that date sugar is less sweet than other natural sweeteners and tastes like dates.

Date sugar can be substituted for sugar in baking and works well in desserts, such as cakes, muffins, and cookies. However, date sugar does not melt well, so blend thoroughly to avoid clumps.

Medjool Dates

Dates are a super fruit, ranking high in antioxidants. Yet, they differ in nutrition from date sugar, as the processing to turn dates into sugar removes nutrition and raises the glycemic index.

Dates are loaded with dietary fiber and often categorized as a laxative food. High levels of soluble fiber are essential in promoting healthy elimination and the comfortable passage of food through the intestinal tract, relieving constipation. To use as a laxative, dates should be soaked overnight, and then eaten in the morning.

These delicious delights contain high levels of minerals, making them a superfood. They strengthen bones and fight off debilitating diseases like osteoporosis. Dates contain selenium, manganese, copper, and magnesium, all of which are important in the development of osteopath cells, which increase bone mineral density and strength.

Breaking Down Dates

First and foremost, dates are easily digested and assimilated, allowing your body to make full use of all their goodness. Dates are loaded with antioxidants, vitamins, minerals, and health-benefiting phytonutrients, making them a powerhouse fruit. The dietary fiber in dates helps to move waste smoothly through your colon, keeping you regular.

Dates contain high levels of iron, a component in hemoglobin in red blood cells that determines the balance of oxygen in the blood. Dates are also high in potassium, an electrolyte that helps control your heart rate and blood pressure.

In addition to iron and potassium, dates contain:

- Carotenes lutein and zeaxanthin
- Copper
- Magnesium
- Manganese
- Vitamin B6
- Niacin
- Pantothenic acid
- Riboflavin

This super fruit is rich in heart healthy nutrients, making dates a fantastic snack for cardiovascular disease-prevention.

Dates are wonderful for sweetening desserts, added in oatmeal, blended in smoothies, or just eaten plain. I enjoy them in my hot and cold foods as a natural and healthy source of fiber and sweetener.

Now that you are an expert in the different types of sweeteners, please take a break from reading and treat yourself to my easy raw cacao truffles sweetened with Medjool dates, but please, don't forget to remove the pits.

Raw Cacao Truffles

Ingredients:
1 cup shredded organic coconut
1 cup raw organic almonds
1 dozen pitted Medjool organic dates

4 tablespoons raw cashew butter
4 tablespoons raw cacao
1½ tablespoons of raw extra virgin coconut oil
1 pinch of Celtic or Himalayan salt
1½ teaspoon organic vanilla extract

Be sure to use raw organic ingredients. Raw cacao is a must. Do *not* use cocoa powder. Cocoa is not raw and is highly processed, making it less nutritious.

Start by putting the almonds and coconut in a food processor and blend for a minute or two, until flour starts to form. Then add the cashew butter, vanilla, Celtic salt, coconut oil, and cacao. Blend for a few seconds before slowly adding the dates.

Continue to blend until everything combines to form a sticky mixture. This mixture can then be rolled into balls and covered in more coconut by rolling them in the shredded coconut. Place the balls in the freezer on wax paper to firm up for an hour or longer, or eat the mixture straight from the food processor.

Keep the remaining balls stored in an airtight container in the refrigerator, if there are any left over. Either way you'll love it!

Suggestion: Double or triple ingredients for more cacao balls, because they are difficult to keep around.

The best sources of unrefined salts and sweeteners can be found in the resource section of this book.

CHAPTER FOURTEEN

Superfoods

And God said, Behold, I have given you every herb-bearing plant which is upon the face of all the earth, and every tree, in the which is the fruit of a tree yielding seed; to you it shall be for meat.

—Genesis 1:29 KJV

What makes superfoods *super*? Superfoods are *superior* foods, nutrient-dense powerhouses that pack large doses of antioxidants, polyphenols, vitamins, and minerals. There is no legal or medical definition for superfoods; they are foods considered to be beneficial for extraordinary health and well-being. Eating them may reduce the risk of chronic disease and increase longevity. People who eat more of them are healthier and more physically fit than those who don't. Superfoods are some of my favorite foods on the planet.

Our Insurance Policy

Did you know that the cure for all sickness has been around longer than the cause?

Real medicines found in superfoods are the medicines that heal, not prescription drugs. The body doesn't have a deficiency of prescription drugs, causing it to be sick. Even those who eat a 100 percent organic diet find it's not always enough. We also need nature-made medicine in the form of superfoods as our insurance policy for extraordinary health.

God wants us to live our lives abundantly, not brokenly. Between the Standard American Diet (SAD) and lab-created prescription drugs, we are not living longer; we are dying longer.

The medicines used in ancient and biblical times were not prescription drugs; they were God-made *adaptogenic* plants. An adaptogen is "a nontoxic substance and especially a plant extract that is held to increase the body's ability to resist the damaging effects of stress and promote or restore normal physiological functioning" (Merriam-Webster, 2016). Adaptogenic herbs are medicine designed perfectly by nature.

> *When diet is incorrect, prescription drugs are of no use.*
> *When diet is correct, prescription drugs are of no need.*
> — Ayurvedic proverb

Naturopathic Medicine

Naturopathic medicine is exactly how real medicine should be, and only God can create such medicine as this. Naturopathic medicine approaches health through the whole person, their lifestyle, and their innate ability to heal. It more often relies on the use of nutrition and therapies that support the body's ability to maintain and achieve wellness without the use of pharmaceuticals.

Modern medicine—known as *allopathic medicine,* including prescription drugs—causes a host of health issues, including blood clots, cancer, and even death. Adaptogenic herbs adapt to our bodies' biological needs that differ from one person to another. There is no one-size-fits-all to healing.

We Must Stop Battling Disease and Start Building Wellness

I believe that we all have a nutritionist living right inside of us, given to us by our loving God. We have an amazing healing mechanism called the immune system, our first line of defense against disease. Removing or *treating* the symptom doesn't address the cause. The causes of sickness are toxicity and deficiency created by a compromised immune system. Removing a lump or a bump or the *symptom* doesn't stop the reason for the sickness. Therefore, a new lump or bump will show its ugly face somewhere else. I call this focus on the symptoms *battling disease.*

Nothing can come close to the infinite healing wisdom of organic foods, raw foods, wild foods, herbal medicines, and adaptogens as super herbs. Plant-based approaches to health challenges are increasing every day at a skyrocketing rate because they work. I proudly announce that we are nearing a critical mass of humans who are shifting their energy and financial power away from a bankrupt, misdirected, environmentally destructive pharmaceutical model of a sick-care industry to a sustainable, preventative, increasing longevity, health-building, self-responsible model of wellness. Super herbs are likely our best allies in this global healing movement.

Incurable Means to Cure From Within

If you listen carefully to the LORD your God and do what is right in his eyes, if you pay attention to his commands and keep all his decrees, I will not bring on you any of the diseases I brought on the Egyptians, for I am the LORD, who heals you.

—Exodus 15:26 NIV

The Earth provides an abundance of perfect foods, and superfoods are superior to any other foods on the planet. Superfoods are nature's medicine and should comprise at least 50 percent of your daily food intake. There are many wonderful superfoods and super herbs provided by nature.

The term *herb* also has more than one definition. Herbs are a small, seed-bearing plant with fleshy, rather than woody, parts. In general, herbs are any plants used for food, flavoring, medicine, or perfume. Culinary use typically distinguishes herbs from spices. Super herbs are tonics that use the power of roots, extracts, berries, bark, and leaves to enhance immunological healing and increase longevity.

Superfoods and Herbs

Multiple lists of superfoods exist across the web and throughout naturopathic healing communities. My list contains superfoods and super herbs.

1. **Cacao** (Raw Chocolate) is the seed/nut of a fruit of an Amazonian tree and the highest antioxidant food on our planet. It provides magnesium, iron, manganese, and chromium. It contains phenylethylamine, theobromine, and anandamide.

This combination is known as the *bliss* chemical.

Raw chocolate:

- Improves cardiovascular health
- Builds strong bones and teeth
- Is a natural aphrodisiac
- Elevates mood
- Increases longevity

Chocolate is truly the food for lovers. I believe that no one is truly allergic to chocolate; it is the processing that makes this healing food allergenic. Aren't you happy now?

2. Goji berries are one of my personal favorites. They have been used in Chinese medicine for more than five thousand years. Also known as the *wolfberry*, Goji berries contain:

- Eighteen kinds of amino acids
- Twenty-one trace minerals
- Antioxidants
- Iron
- Polysaccharides
- B and E vitamins

They provide the necessary energy to handle just about any difficulty. Traditionally, it is believed that constant consumption of Goji will instill a cheerful attitude, and there's nothing like good cheer to overcome stress.

Goji berries are also considered brain food. They are full of antioxidants that help protect against neuro-degenerative disorders like Alzheimer's disease and oxidative stress in the brain. Goji berries increase longevity, strength, and overall well-being.

3. Maca is a Peruvian radish. This adaptogenic superfood increases energy, endurance, strength, and libido. It has been a staple food in the Peruvian Andes for thousands of years. Maca works on a cellular level, enhancing and balancing hormones to an optimal level. Dried maca powder contains more than 10 percent protein and nearly twenty amino acids. This radish contains five times more protein and four times more fiber than a potato (Wolfe, 2013).

4. Hemp seeds are packed with nutrients. They contain iron, amino acids, vitamin E, and are 33 percent digestible protein. Gamma linolenic acid (GLA) is a fatty substance found in various plant seed oils, such as hemp oil, making it an effective medicine for skin conditions, such as psoriasis and eczema. Hemp is loaded with omega-3s, which are important for inflammation reduction, cell regeneration, and healthy brain function.

5. Bee products such as totally raw, organic honey in its organic, wild, unfiltered form is similar to a multivitamin. Bee pollen contains nearly all B vitamins and all twenty-one essential amino acids, making it a complete protein. This superior food is abundant in minerals, antioxidants, probiotics, and enzymes.

6. Camu Berry the fruit of the camu camu shrub is packed with more vitamin C than any other food on the planet. It rebuilds tissue, purifies the blood, and enhances immunity. Camu berry modulates the immune system and is a natural antidepressant. It also has eye-nourishing properties. Camu berry is one of the top superfoods in the world.

7. Sea Vegetables (kelp, dulse, nori, hijiki, bladder wrack, spirulina, and chlorella) benefit the entire body by:

- Helping remove heavy metals
- Detoxifying the body
- Providing numerous trace minerals
- Regulating immunity
- Decreasing the risk of cancer
- Regulating blood pressure
- Balancing blood glucose levels

They support the thyroid, immune system, adrenals, and hormone function. I consider sea vegetables to be one of nature's most complete food sources, providing optimal calcium, blood oxygenation, and a complete protein.

8. Medicinal Mushrooms (cordyceps, maitake, shiitake, lion's mane, chaga) are super immune-enhancing compounds. Mushrooms contain some of the most potent natural substances on the planet, which is why they deliver a tremendous boost to your immune system. Medicinal mushrooms are one of the most intelligent adaptogenic superfoods on the planet. They have proven effective in healing cancer and a variety of other ailments (Wolfe, 2013).

Chaga is known as the king of the medicinal mushrooms and is literally considered a gift from God. Chaga is powerful, because it contains the nutrients and the force of actual trees. Tree mushrooms contain some of the most potent natural medicines on the planet. Some trees live ten thousand years or more, making these mushrooms the most powerful living beings in the world. Of the one hundred forty thousand species of mushroom-forming fungi, science is familiar with only 10 percent, according to world-renown mycologist Paul Stamets, who has written six books on the topic. I highly suggest that you extend your research and read Paul Stamets' book collection, available at major booksellers.

9. Noni is a small evergreen tree in the Pacific islands. Its fruit's many health benefits may be exactly what you need to alleviate pain. *Scopoletin*, found in noni, is a naturally occurring, powerful pain relieving constituent.

Other benefits of noni include:

- Prevents cancer
- Promotes healthy liver function
- Maintains cardiovascular health
- Relaxes muscles
- Soothes psoriasis and eczema
- Relieves memory problems
- Supports immune health

In addition, the antioxidant levels in raw noni juice provide antipsychotic, antifungal, antibacterial, and anti-inflammatory effects that aid in treatments for arthritis and disorders related to central nervous system.

10. Astragalus is a natural dietary supplement used for various health conditions. For instance, it's used to treat the common cold, upper respiratory infections, fibromyalgia, and diabetes. In traditional Chinese medicine, astragalus is known for its disease-fighting properties. Astragalus has been used successfully for thousands of years to combat stress and reverse disease.

11. Turmeric is an orange-colored spice imported from India. It is part of the ginger family and has been used in Middle Eastern and Southeast Asian cooking for thousands of years.

In addition, Ayurvedic and Chinese medicines use turmeric to clear infections and inflammations on the inside and outside of the body. Western medical practitioners have only recently come on board in recognizing the health benefits of turmeric.

12. Curcumin, the main component in turmeric, is a substance with powerful anti-inflammatory and high antioxidant properties and appears to block an enzyme that promotes the growth of head and neck cancer. Curcumin has been found to stop the spread of malignant cells. Turmeric has powerful antioxidant properties that fight cancer-causing free radicals, reducing or preventing the damage they have the potential to cause.

13. Holy Basil is a super herb also known as *Tulsi*. It is a member of the sweet basil family, yet a member of the mint family. Holy basil is used for many stress-related ailments, such as anxiety and depression. Tulsi also has medicinal prosperities that work successfully with heart distress and respiratory disorders.

14. Schizandra Berry although a berry, it is a major adaptogenic Chinese herb. Schizandra helps keep you relaxed and alert and supports the central nervous system. Schizandra is considered one of the premium mind tonics of herbalism. It is used to support concentration, memory, and alertness.

When I first sipped a cup of Schizandra berry tea, I could not figure out the taste—in fact, I tasted five different flavors. In traditional Chinese medicine, *Wu Wei Zi* means *of five different flavors*: sweet, sour, salty, bitter, and pungent, exactly my own personal experience. Schizandra, unlike caffeinated beverages, does not produce nervousness. It is mildly *calming* while producing wakefulness and mental focus. If you're feeling anxious, schizandra will calm you down. If you're feeling low, schizandra will lift you up, without the jitters.

15. Reishi Mushroom is the perfect super-adaptogen herb for modern times. It is known as the *queen of the medicinal mushrooms*. Reishi is strengthening, protective, and calming to the nerves. It is a potent tonic for both *qi*—vital energy—and for *shen*—spirit. It is the perfect anti-stress herb. It helps to center you. When you're consuming Reishi, you feel protected and well-balanced.

16. Matcha Green Tea, an incredible green tea, is an antioxidant-rich powerhouse beverage made famous by Japanese tea ceremonies for more than nine hundred years.

Matcha tea:

- Fights cancer
- Burns fat
- Reduces anxiety
- Calms the central nervous system
- Improves mental alertness
- Strengthens the immune system

One serving of matcha green tea is the nutritional equivalent of ten cups of regularly brewed green tea. Matcha green tea has one hundred forty times more antioxidants than regularly brewed green tea. These chlorophyll-rich leaves are handpicked, steamed, dried, and ground into a fine green powder, making it a nutrient-rich beverage.

17. Ashwagandha is what I consider to be *the balancing herb*; it boosts the body's supply of antioxidants and regulates the immune system. The immune system is your first line of defense against disease. Ashwagandha is also known as *Indian ginseng* and has a wide range of other health benefits, including the reduction of inflammation, arthritis, asthma, hypertension, stress, and rheumatism. This extremely powerful super herb has the ability to fight cancer and diabetes. I use ashwagandha as part of my daily nutritional regimen.

18. Avocados are high in potassium. They support healthy blood pressure and blood glucose levels, making avocados an ideal food. Avocados contain 100 percent monounsaturated fatty acids, making them a highly nutritious fruit that produces a healthy oil. Eighty percent of the calories in avocados are from fat, making it one of the fattiest plant foods in existence.

Ok, you can stop screaming now. The right fats, such as avocados, do not make you fat. As a matter of fact, the fat in avocados is called *oleic acid*, which has been known to reduce inflammation and has beneficial effects on genes linked to cancer and obesity. Avocados improve your metabolic system by triggering hormones that release fat. Yes, I am saying that avocados are great for weight loss.

Did you know that avocados help shed unwanted birth weight, prevent cervical cancers, balance hormones, and increase fertility? It takes nine months for an avocado to blossom into a ripened fruit, the same time it takes a fetus to grow into a baby.

Now that you have a general idea of the science behind the scenes of nature's medicine chest, let's define medicine: *Medicine is a superior food made preferably of plants that creates balance, serenity, calmness, and overall healing within the body.*

Plant medicine is a form of healing that considers the whole person, body, mind, spirit, and emotions in the quest for optimal health and wellness.

> *Let food be thy medicine and medicine be thy food.*
> —Hippocrates

The best sources for superfoods and super herbs can be found in the resource section of this book.

CHAPTER FIFTEEN

Juicing and Blending

As a holistic practitioner, I get asked this common question all the time: which is better — juicing or blending?

First and foremost, one is not better than the other. Blending is the process of thoroughly blending whole fruits and vegetables into a smoothie. Smoothies are created in blenders and include the produce's fiber. Juicing is the process of extracting the liquid content of whole foods through a special juicing machine. Most of the fiber is then discarded or used as compost.

Both juicing and blending are beneficial, but in different ways. Juicing extracts the nutrients from produce and discards the indigestible fiber. By removing fiber, your digestive system doesn't have to work as hard to break down the food and absorb the nutrients. Juicing is like intravenous therapy, traveling directly into your bloodstream for rapid delivery of vital nutrients. In fact, the nutrients are more readily available to the body in larger quantities than if you were to eat the fruits and vegetables whole.

I consider juicing a rapid, life-force delivery of enzymes and critical nutrients, surpassing digestion. Juicing requires only about 4 percent of your digestion process. It is a great way to receive an abundance of minerals, nutrients, and enzymes without work.

Why are we removing the fiber; don't we need it?

Fiber provides energy, keeps us full, regulates digestion, and creates healthy stool formation. However, for rapid healing and detox, it is best to remove the fiber in favor of a rapid delivery of nutrients. Juicing is helpful for patients who have chronic health conditions and those with severe digestive disorders.

Most people today suffer impaired digestion from less-than-optimal food choices over many years. If you suffer digestive issues, your body's ability to absorb all the nutrients from vegetables is limited. Juicing helps to *pre-digest* them for you, so you will receive most of the nutrition, rather than wasting nutrients in elimination.

JUICING

Juicing Is the Key to Radiant Skin

Pardon me if I sound modest, but people ask me all the time what I use on my skin. I tell them that healthy, glowing skin comes from within.

Freshly juiced vegetables are a healing and detoxifying modality. Juicing is nutrient-dense and therefore nourishes and restores the body at a cellular level. The aftermath of a fresh raw juice creates an illuminating instant glow. The accumulative effect of daily juicing will surpass those expensive skin creams, because great skin comes from within. That rapid, life-force delivery of vital nutrients protects the body against cellular, oxidative stress called *accelerated aging*. Raw juicing is high in zinc, C, and E, which are known to promote healthy, supple skin.

The biggest health advantage of juicing is *cellular cleansing*. Juicing cleanses our outsides better and faster than any skin care line. Juicing is extremely easy on our digestive systems and travels into our systems rapidly because it is only using 4 percent of our digestion. Fresh raw juices also combat skin disorders.

Juicing is great for the liver. Experts say there are well over eight hundred duties of the liver. Therefore, eliminating toxins is of great help to your liver. Juicing pushes nutrients through your bloodstream, into your liver, and expels toxins out of your body. The result: a healthful glow.

Blood Sugar

When you remove fiber from produce, the liquid juice is absorbed quickly into your bloodstream. If you juice only fruits or high-sugar content vegetables like carrots and beets, you may experience a rapid spike in blood sugar and fluctuating blood glucose levels. This imbalance can lead to mood swings, dizziness, weakness, and energy loss.

Lemons and limes are the exception to this rule; they have virtually none of the offending sugar and fructose responsible for metabolic disturbances. Additionally, lemons or limes eliminate the bitter taste of the dark, deep green leafy vegetables that provide most of the benefits of juicing. Adding one small, green apple with the skin is also a great way to please your palette without a blood sugar spike.

The Best Time to Juice

I'm not going to lie to you; juicing can be time consuming. Many people ask me if they can make juice first thing in the morning, and then drink it later. This is not a good idea. Vegetable juice is highly perishable, so it's best to drink it immediately or within twenty minutes after making it. If you're careful, you can store it twenty-four hours in a tightly sealed mason jar but only moderate nutrition will remain.

Is it helpful at all to bring your juice to work so you can consume it during the day?

If you have no other choice but to make your juice in advance, pour your juice in a glass mason jar with an airtight lid. Fill it to the *very* top. Leave minimal air in the jar. Air causes oxidization that destroys the nutrients and damages the juice.

Immediately store the jar in the refrigerator and consume it when you are ready. It is best to drink your juice as soon as possible. However, even if you are storing it correctly, do not store it any longer than twenty-four hours.

I juice in the morning, a great way to break my fast. If that does not work out well for your busy schedule, please feel free to choose whatever works best for your lifestyle. I recommend storing juice rather than avoiding juicing due to a lack of time.

Cleaning Your Juicer

First, a juicer takes longer than a few minutes to clean and most people will use this as an excuse not to juice at all. Most juicers come with a brush for cleaning the metal blade. Now if your juicer does not come with a brush, I find that using an old toothbrush works well on the metal grater. Always clean your juicer immediately after you juice to prevent any remnants from contaminating the juicer with mold growth.

If you buy a decent, high-quality juicer, the entire process should only take about five minutes. I juice every morning and it only takes me five to seven minutes to wash my produce, make my juice, and clean the juicer. It's not bad at all. In my opinion, fresh raw juice is an amazing, healing drink that is worth the time and the added effort.

Aren't you worth it?

I know I am, and I believe you certainly are, too.

Juice Is NOT a Meal

Although there are many benefits of juicing, realize that juice has very little protein and virtually no fat. It is not a complete food by itself. It should be used in addition to your regular meals and not as a meal substitute. Unless you are on a special detoxification program, it is not wise to use juicing as a meal replacement. Juicing can safely be consumed in between meals or as a temporary fasting break to cleanse and rest the organs, supervised under the care of a qualified practitioner.

BLENDING

Blender Shakes

Smoothies, on the other hand, are a fantastic meal replacement. They include fiber and are a great lunch to take with you on the go or to work. I enjoy a smoothie every single day because it gives me control. I choose the foods and give myself a nutrient-dense, powerhouse shake to get me through my afternoon. I do not have to *reheat* a meal, plus I can avoid a typical lunch of processed meats and refined grain breads that leave the body bloated and tired.

Getting the right amount of fruits and vegetables our bodies require can sometimes be a challenge. Smoothies are a great way to receive the daily requirements of fruits and vegetables packed into a creamy and delicious dessert. Blending a couple of servings of each into a smoothie helps ensure that you meet your body's daily nutritional needs.

Smoothies

Making your own nutrient-dense smoothie doesn't take as much time as preparing most meals, freeing time for other things. Taking a smoothie with you is convenient, helping you to avoid grabbing an unhealthy choice.

Smoothies contain essential vitamins and minerals and are an easy way to nourish your body. The best way to know the exact ingredients in your smoothie is to make your own. Freshly made smoothies give you the control of what's in them rather than purchasing the already made versions that may contain processed sugars and unwanted ingredients that you can surely do without.

Kids Love Them

Getting our children to eat healthy foods is not always easy. I know firsthand what that's like with my daughter, Michaela. Fortunately, most kids love the taste of a creamy smoothie, naturally sweetened by fruit and or a good sweetener like raw honey, maple syrup, dates, or pure green leaf stevia. You can even hide veggies in your kids' smoothies that they won't even know are there.

SHHH! I won't say anything—this can be our little secret.

Other Benefits of Smoothies

Drinking smoothies can satisfy your hunger and help you reach your goal weight as well as the required intake of fiber. Men need approximately thirty-eight grams of fiber per day; women should consume twenty-five grams. One serving of fruit typically contains two to four grams of fiber. The highest concentration of fiber is found in apples, blackberries, and pears—five to seven grams per serving. Fruit's soluble fiber slows digestion and helps control blood glucose levels, lowering your risk of diabetes.

As I write this, I am craving my next smoothie, especially after seeing the benefits in black and white. Taking care of my body is one of my highest priorities. Another priority is extending this life-changing information to you.

I hope that I ignited a fire within you to begin juicing daily for the rapid delivery of healing nutrients and enzymes. I hope you can't wait to blend your next meal with nutrient-rich fruits and veggies.

RECIPES

Here are some of my wonderful raw juice recipes. Kids will love them, too. Organic ingredients are a must for optimal flavor and nutritional value. Remember that genetic mutations and chemical fertilizers deplete soil and deplete nutrients. Be creative with your juices, as these recipes can be followed as is or used as guides to create your own.

Drink daily and be creative.

The Refresher

4 kale leaves
1 whole cucumber with skin
1 lemon with skin
1 apple with skin
4 stalks celery
1 small beet

The Spa

5 romaine leaves
1 whole cucumber with skin
1 lemon with skin
1 apple with skin
4 stalks celery
1 small beet
2 large carrots

The Happy Apple

1 bunch of parsley
4 kale leaves
1 whole cucumber with skin
1 lemon with skin
1 apple with skin
4 stalks celery
1 small beet

The Energizer

4 kale leaves
1 zucchini with skin
1 lemon with skin

4 celery stalks
1 apple with skin

The Vitalizer

1 lime with skin
4 celery stalks
A bunch of spinach
1 cucumber with skin
1 bunch cilantro
1 apple with skin

The Eye Opener

4 large carrots
1 zucchini with skin
1 lemon with skin
1 apple with skin
4 celery stalks
1 bunch cilantro

The Digestive Aid

1 apple with skin
1 knuckle ginger
1 cucumber
3 celery stalks
1 green lime with skin
1 stalk fennel
1 bunch romaine

Here are some of my delicious smoothie recipes that I've created for you. Use organic ingredients to avoid chemical fertilizers, which can be harmful to your health. The kids will enjoy these like a dessert, not realizing they are drinking something healthy.

Raspberry Avocado Smoothie

> 1 cup frozen organic raspberries
> 1 ripe organic avocado
> ½ organic ripe banana
> ½ teaspoon raw organic honey
> 1 cup whole plain organic yogurt
> 1 tablespoon organic, extra virgin coconut oil
> ½ teaspoon vanilla extract

Blend and enjoy!

Chocolate Avocado Smoothie

> 1 medium cold ripe organic banana
> 2 tablespoons raw cacao powder
> ½ ripe organic avocado
> ½ cup plain yogurt
> 1 teaspoon raw honey
> ½ teaspoon organic vanilla extract
> 1 tablespoon organic, extra virgin coconut oil

Blend and enjoy!

Berry Delicious Smoothie

> 1 cup frozen mixed organic berries
> ½ cup organic full-fat organic coconut milk
> Coconut milk (canned is fine)
> 1 teaspoon raw honey
> 1 organic banana
> 1 tablespoon organic almond butter
> 1 tablespoon organic, extra virgin coconut oil

Blend and enjoy!

Powerhouse Smoothie

½ cup frozen organic peaches
1½ banana
1½ cup raw cow milk or goat kefir (plain & whole)
1 tablespoon organic flax oil
1 tablespoon raw honey
1 heaping teaspoon organic, extra virgin coconut oil
A few dashes of cinnamon

Blend and enjoy!

Piña Colada Smoothie

½ cup fresh or frozen organic pineapple
2 tablespoons frozen coconut meat or coconut butter
1 teaspoon organic, extra virgin coconut oil
1 teaspoon vanilla extract
6 ounces of coconut water
1 teaspoon raw honey

Blend and enjoy!

Tropical Paradise

1 cup raw coconut water (Harmless Harvest)
½ cup frozen or fresh mango
½ cup pineapple
½ banana
A few strawberries
1 tablespoon raw honey
1 teaspoon organic, extra virgin coconut oil
1 teaspoon raw coconut butter

Blend and enjoy!

Almond Joy Smoothie

1 tablespoon raw almond butter
1 teaspoon coconut oil
1 teaspoon raw cacao nibs
6 ounces raw coconut water
1 teaspoon extra virgin, organic coconut oil
½ ripe organic banana
½ teaspoon raw organic honey
1 teaspoon organic vanilla extract

Blend and enjoy!

Pumpkin Pie Smoothie

1 cup plain whole organic yogurt
¾ cup canned organic pumpkin, chilled
½ cup ice cubes
1 teaspoon raw organic honey
½ teaspoon ground organic cinnamon
¼ teaspoon ground organic nutmeg
1 ripe organic banana
1 teaspoon organic vanilla extract
1 teaspoon organic, extra virgin coconut oil

Blend and enjoy!

Blueberry Dream Smoothie

1 cup organic fresh or frozen blueberries
1 cup plain whole organic yogurt or kefir
1 tablespoon extra virgin coconut oil
1 teaspoon raw organic honey

1 teaspoon flaxseed oil
½ ripe organic banana

Blend and enjoy!

Banana Muffin Smoothie

1 ripe banana
1 teaspoon organic extra virgin coconut oil
1 teaspoon organic vanilla extract
½ teaspoon organic cinnamon
1 handful raw, organic walnuts (approx. 6 nuts)
1 teaspoon raw organic honey
1 cup plain whole organic yogurt
½ teaspoon organic maple syrup

Blend and enjoy!

Protein Powerhouse Smoothie

1 cup goat milk kefir
½ teaspoon organic vanilla extract
I cup mixed frozen organic berries
1 teaspoon organic cinnamon
1 tablespoon organic, extra virgin coconut oil
½ ripe organic banana
1 tablespoon hemp seeds
1 tablespoon organic almond butter

Blend and enjoy!

HIGH Protein Power House Smoothie

> 1 tablespoon raw almond butter
> 1 teaspoon flaxseed oil
> 1 teaspoon organic, extra virgin coconut oil
> 1 teaspoon raw bee pollen granules
> 1 cup plain goat kefir
> 1 teaspoon raw organic honey
> 1 whole ripe organic banana
> ½ cup mixed fresh or frozen organic berries

Blend and enjoy!

Amazing Green Machine

> 1 cut green apple
> 2 sticks celery
> ½ avocado
> ½ cucumber with skin
> 2 handfuls of spinach, kale, or romaine
> 1 banana
> 5–7 dates
> 1 cup raw coconut water

Blend and enjoy!

The Refresher Smoothie

> 1 lemon, peeled
> 1 cucumber, peeled and chopped
> 1 banana, peeled
> 1 apple, peeled, cored, and chopped
> 1 bunch of cilantro
> 1 bunch of kale

½ cup water
4 pitted dates
½ cup ice
½ cup raw coconut water

Blend and enjoy!

Your health is relying on the sources you choose. The best sources for juicers and blenders are listed in the resource section of this book.

CHAPTER SIXTEEN

Healing Modalities

Although I do encourage whole, organic, God-made food sources, the body doesn't only depend on the food that we eat to remain healthy. There are other modalities that greatly affect our health. Here are the healing modalities that I incorporate into my health regimen, and I encourage you do the same.

Intermittent Fasting

> *Go gather together all the Jews who are in Susa, and fast for me. Do not eat or drink for three days, night or day. I and my attendants will fast as you do. When it is done, I will go to the king, even though it isn't the law. And if I perish, I perish.*
>
> —Esther 4:16 NIV

Consuming healthy, God-made, whole, organic foods are the Almighty Physician's recommendations for optimal health. Partial fasting, also known as intermittent fasting, is an additional recommendation in God's healing modalities. To successfully heal the body, we must at times abstain from food even when we are hungry. Intermittent fasting involves skipping meals during a specific period during the day, and then returning to your normal schedule of healthy food.

Intermittent *fasting* is a partial fast that heals the body of various health conditions and leads to extraordinary health. A partial fast could be from 1:30 p.m. to 7:30 p.m. or from 5:30 p.m. until noon the next day. Your intermittent fasting time should be at least four hours of wake time in addition to your fasting sleep hours. It takes approximately six to eight hours for your body to burn all sugar out of your system.

Breakfast is not the most important meal of the day.

I begin every morning with 16 ounces of pure, clean water and 1 tablespoon of raw apple cider vinegar. Then, I refrain from all food until midday. I drink raw, homemade juice with added super herbs and other nutrient-rich superfoods all in their raw, live form to break my fast.

Intermittent fasting allows the body's organs to rest and heal. Restricting the body from caloric intake provides many health benefits, which include:

- Better digestion
- Healthy, glowing skin
- Alleviated pain
- Healthy weight loss
- Relief from gas and bloating
- Rejuvenated organ function
- Reduced inflammation
- Reduced oxidative stress
- Increased capacity to cope with stress

In addition, intermittent fasting clears the mind and helps us to connect and hear from God.

I ate no pleasant bread, neither came flesh nor wine to my mouth, neither did I anoint myself at all, till three whole weeks were fulfilled.

—Daniel 10:3 KJV

Earthing and Grounding

The practice of *earthing* or *grounding* requires your body to have direct contact with the Earth's surface energy by walking, sitting, or sleeping outside. When we contact the Earth directly through touch, our bodies become saturated with negative ions and free electrons. We are equalized to the same electric energy level as the Earth.

Historically, humans have spent more time outdoors and touched the Earth much more than modern humans. We had direct contact with the soil, from walking on the ground barefoot. Today we wear rubber shoes, are exposed to electric magnetic fields (EMFs) daily, and don't often come into direct contact with the ground.

We ground electrical outlets to avoid the buildup of excess positive charge. Our bodies need the same type of grounding, because we are electric too.

Here are some of the many health attributes from earthing and grounding:

- Reduction of inflammation by defusing excess positive electrons
- Reduction of chronic pain
- Improved sleep
- Normalized biological rhythms, including circadian rhythm

- Increased energy
- Lower stress levels
- Improved blood pressure and blood flow
- Balanced hormones
- Adrenal health
- Relief from muscle tension and headaches
- Feelings of balance and serenity

So be sure to remove your shoes and enjoy direct contact with the energy of the Earth (wellnessmama.com).

Sun Gazing

Sun gazing is the act of looking directly into the sun, often as part of a spiritual or religious practice. However, the human eye is very sensitive, and exposure to direct sunlight can lead to solar retinopathy, so you should always limit the time spent sun gazing. I have learned that sun gazing can be done once every ten months with caution by starting with only a few seconds and working your way up, not to exceed forty seconds. However, I believe, despite what I have read and tried, that sun gazing is not for everyone, and one should take caution.

The practice of sun gazing has been used as a healing therapy for centuries. The sun is the basis of all life, and without it we would die. Staring at the sun can infuse the body with large amounts of energy at sunrise and or sunset, when the sun is closest to the Earth. Sun gazers stand barefoot on the Earth and look directly at the sun for ten seconds. Every day, ten seconds are added and some sun gazers eventually reach a duration of forty-four minutes, which I would not recommend.

Research has shown that sun gazing has many health benefits. It boosts the production of the feel-good hormones—serotonin, dopamine, and melatonin. Sun gazing also increases energy, improves eyesight, and delivers a sense of balance.

Sun gazing should be practiced when the sun is going down or early in the morning when the sun is less intense. If you have never sun gazed, begin before sunset or during sunrise on a day when the sun is obstructed by clouds. You can then increase your sessions gradually as you would sunbathing, exercising, or anything else for that matter. Please keep in mind that if you do too much, you may harm yourself.

Sun Protection Comes From Within

Please do not be afraid of the sun: the sun gives life force and energy and does not cause cancer. The sun has received a bad rap for decades, because a tan is one of the best forms of sunscreen you can have.

The sun has evolved for centuries, since the inception of time. Lack of sun exposure causes deficiencies and sickness. The use of chemical-laden, carcinogenic sunscreens is the root cause of many cancers. Most sunscreen lotions on the market have ingredients that are a direct cause of most cancers. Yet, we are promoting them as a healthy alternative to the sun.

Sun protection starts from within—a diet high in antioxidants of real, organic, God-made whole foods. My skin used to burn in the sun, even though I am of Italian descent. I believe my previous diet was the culprit. However, my current diet of whole, organic, high quality nutrition has proved differently. Now, I sun bathe without any sun block and never burn. I am not saying that this is wise for everyone, especially if their diet is insufficient in the nutrients needed for proper protection.

Sunburn is a type of inflammation, and your diet is the root cause. By slathering on chemical-laden sunscreens, you will not prevent skin cancer. You may increase your chances of developing it. Eating a diet of healthy fats like avocados, coconut products, and high antioxidant-rich foods such as berries, raw nuts, leafy greens, and raw cacao can increase your body's natural skin protectors and also support other areas of health.

Our bodies generate vitamin D from the sun's rays. The ultraviolet rays and our skin combine to convert the sun's rays into vitamin D. Over the past few decades, an overwhelming number of people have become deficient in this vital nutrient and are suffering enormous consequences. More people are dying every year from health issues concerning vitamin D deficiencies. This massive deficiency is a result of avoiding the sun, in addition to the SAD (Standard American Diet). The sun can prevent skin cancer, breast cancer, prostate cancer, bladder cancer — almost every type of cancer. The sun can also prevent autoimmune and other immunological diseases.

Studies reveal that people with melanoma who previously had frequent sun exposure had improved survival rates over those who avoided the sun. One such study was conducted by the *European Journal of Cancer* (Rosso, 2008). Now, if previous sun exposure helped those with melanoma survive, then how did they get cancer in the first place? Great question, because the sun doesn't cause cancer.

The real causes of cancer and other diseases have been explained in this book. I hope you will not blame the sun.

Oil Pulling

The oral health practices of Ayurveda include *oil pulling* as a healing modality. Oil pulling uses coconut oil to prevent bleeding gums, decay, dryness of throat, oral malodor, cracked and dry lips and for strengthening teeth, gums, and the jaw. Oil pulling removes toxins from the body through the swishing process, which draws oral and bodily poisons. This modality is one of the best ways to remove bacteria and promote healthy teeth and gums. Coconut oil is the recommended for oil pulling due to its antifungal, antiviral, and antiparasitic compounds.

Oil pulling:

- Kills bad breath
- Heals bleeding gums
- Whitens teeth
- Prevents cavities
- Soothes throat dryness
- Prevents heart disease
- Reduces inflammation
- Improves acne
- Boosts immune function

Oil pulling detoxifies the oral cavity like soap removes dirt. Oil pulling draws the toxins out of your mouth and creates a clean, antiseptic oral environment that contributes to the natural flow of oral liquids that are necessary for the prevention of tooth decay, cavities, and gum disease.

Instructions: The best time for this procedure is first thing the morning before you drink or eat anything. Your mouth will have a full presence of bacteria.

Gently swish 1 tablespoon of coconut oil around your mouth and teeth for approximately 15–20 minutes.

Do not swallow the oil since there is now bacteria present in the oil.

After the 20 minutes, spit the oil into the trash. Spitting into a sink or toilet will clog your plumbing.

Rinse your mouth thoroughly and brush immediately.

Repeat this procedure every day or 3–4 times per week for optimal oral and physical health benefits.

Dry Brushing

Did you know that one third of your body's toxins are excreted through the skin and dry brushing helps to unclog pores and excrete toxins that are trapped in your skin?

Your skin plays a large role in supporting optimal detoxification. *Dry skin brushing* can be a valuable tool to remove dead skin cells and activate waste removal from your lymph nodes. Dry brushing is a modality that I use every day before I shower.

Lymph means a pure clean stream and dry brushing helps keep the lymphatic system clean. Your skin is a complex system made up of nerves, glands, and cell layers that protect your body from extreme temperatures and chemicals. Your skin also manufactures antibacterial substances to protect you from infection. By stimulating your lymphatic system through dry brushing, you're removing toxins and dead skin, improving appearance, improving digestion and kidney function, clearing your clogged pores, and allowing your skin to breathe.

Dry brushing also increases circulation, which, in turn, encourages the elimination of toxic waste. This process also softens hard fat deposits located below the skin while evenly distributing fat deposits, which may reduce the appearance of cellulite. Dry brushing increases healthy blood flow and is extremely invigorating and stress relieving.

Instructions: First, choose a natural bristle brush with a long handle. Remove your clothing and brush your skin, starting at your feet and brushing upward in long circular motions toward your heart. Always brush toward your heart. Continue to brush several times in each area, overlapping as you go. Please be careful as you brush over more sensitive areas, like the breasts. Your skin will become less sensitive if you dry brush regularly. Once you've brushed your entire body for about three to four minutes, take your shower. This process stimulates blood circulation, bringing more blood to the top layers of the skin and creating a healthy glow (Jenkins, 2014).

Continue to dry brush your entire body every day. Don't forget to clean your brush with soap and water once a week. Then hang your brush to dry after use to avoid any mildew accumulation that can lead to health problems.

That's right, it's not only our hair and dogs that need brushing; our bodies can benefit as well.

Exercise

Exercise makes you feel better simply because it turns on your inner garbage disposal and helps your body remove toxins. This detox is experienced through sweating. Exercise increases energy and stimulates the feel-good hormones—serotonin and dopamine—putting you in a good mood. This prize-winning healing modality also keeps you fit and healthy by toning muscle mass and burning fat. Exercise also keeps the doctor away since it purifies the blood and keeps your cardiovascular system in optimal shape. Swimming and walking are fun, freeing, and low impact, making them both excellent and popular choices for almost anyone.

Rebounding

Turn on your inner garbage disposal with rebounding. *Rebounding* is an exercise that improves your sense of balance while directly strengthening the immune system. A rebounder is a mini trampoline, allowing you to bounce up and down, resulting in low-impact movement that increases agility. This exercise is extremely effective in stimulating your lymphatic system, which is responsible for the removal of impurities from the bloodstream.

Rebounding reduces body fat while firming your thighs, legs, hips, and abdominal area. I enjoy bouncing on my rebounder while watching my favorite movie, especially when it's too cold to exercise outdoors. Jumping up and down on a rebounder is a beneficial modality in both cleansing and healing.

Massage Therapy

I love what I do, and part of that love is taking optimal care of *me,* so I can take better care of you. Massage therapy is a modality I enjoy often.

Massage therapy is touted as a luxury, yet I believe that massage is a necessity to better health. Massage relaxes the body and relieves stress. It balances hormones which regulate sleep, heartbeat, blood glucose levels, and blood pressure. It protects the brain and nervous system. Massage increases serotonin and dopamine, the feel-good hormones in the brain. It stimulates immune function, our first line of defense against disease. It is amazing how God created us perfectly equipped with every healing tool right inside of us.

> *God created mankind in his own image, in the image of*
> *God he created them; male and female he created them.*
> —Genesis 1:27 ISV

Foot and Hand Reflexology

The feet are a map for the body's organs; the areas located on your feet correspond to organs and systems of your body. *Reflexology* is based on the principle that there are reflexes in the hands and feet that relate to every organ, gland, and system of the body. For example, the stomach and pancreas areas are found in the arch of the foot.

The adrenal gland reflex point is located above the kidney point on the soles of each of your feet. This resembles your anatomy, where an adrenal gland perches atop each kidney. Long-term stress can fatigue the adrenal glands because they're responsible for our *fight or flight* response. Stress causes the adrenals to release adrenaline and cortisol. Reflexology releases those negative responses and increases a sense of well-being and healthy adrenal function.

Most problems within the body *reflect* to the feet and can be diagnosed and treated through foot massage. Reflexology of the hands and feet is a powerful form of preventative medicine, and should be incorporated as part of your regimen.

The benefits of reflexology focus on the reduction of stress. Because the feet and hands help set the tension level for the entire body, they provide easy access to stress signals, allowing them to be interrupted. The massage of these areas can reset *homeostasis*, the body's equilibrium.

Hand reflexology is associated with the fingertips and palms, reflecting the upper part of the head, which includes the brain, sinuses, ears, and eyes. The hands also represent the heart, gallbladder, intestines, and spine.

Your Feet Are Your Second Heart

The feet have a vital job. They move blood flow back into the heart through their veins. The heart constantly constricts and loosens, just like a pump. If you step on the ground and force pressure on the feet, it will help to pump the blood directly back to the heart. The vein itself has valves to prevent the blood from flowing backwards. Foot reflexology and massage help the muscles to tighten and loosen properly, which encourages the valves to function optimally.

Chiropractic Care

The spine is the backbone of your health. Chiropractic care is a system of complementary medicine—a natural form of health care—that uses spinal adjustments to correct misalignments and restore balance within the body. Your spinal column is made up of twenty-four independent vertebrae and allows your body to move and bend through every motion of each day. Your spine also helps protect the central nervous system that controls and coordinates every muscle, ligament, tissue, nerve, and organ of the body.

When vertebrae aren't functioning together properly it is called *misalignment*, or a *subluxation*. These subluxations cause you to experience pain, discomfort, decreased mobility, or joint dysfunctions, creating a malfunction between your brain and body.

Chiropractic care relieves these issues and treats numerous conditions, such as:

- Chronic headaches
- Sinus problems
- High blood pressure
- Ear infections
- Leg pain
- Arthritis
- Fibromyalgia
- Allergies
- Neck injuries

Sex

Do you know the health benefits gained by having sex? Sex can improve your relationship by increasing the hormone level oxytocin, a feel-good hormone elevated during and after an orgasm.

Sex boosts immunity, is great exercise, lowers your risk of developing prostate cancer, and keeps testosterone and estrogen levels in balance. Sex lowers blood pressure, helps with bladder control, and relieves stress. Sex releases pain-reducing hormones, which lessens pain from backaches, arthritis, menstrual cramps, and headaches. Sex improves sleep, creates intimacy, and boosts your libido.

Caution: Practice safe sex to reduce your risk of developing a sexually transmitted disease.

Cleansing and Detoxing

Toxicity and deficiency are the root of most diseases. When toxic, it becomes difficult for the body to absorb valuable nutrients. This problem leads to deficiency. The immune system, our first line of defense against disease, becomes compromised. *Autointoxication*, or self-poisoning, affects billions of people every day. Most of these people are unaware.

Symptoms of autointoxication may include:

- Gas
- Bloating
- Tiredness
- Lack of energy
- Recurring infections
- Allergies
- Asthma
- Irritability
- Mood swings
- Insomnia

Autointoxication may even lead to heart disease and many types of cancer.

Internal cleansing is critical for optimal health. Some of the best ways to limit toxic exposure is to consume mostly organic and unprocessed foods in addition to cooking and living in a minimally toxic environment.

If we diligently follow the principles in this book and cleanse four times a year with the change of the seasons, we greatly enhance our health. Here is an example of a basic, simple cleansing and detox program.

Tonijean's Three-Day, Gentle, Feel-Great Cleanse

In the morning, break your fast and drink 12–16 ounces of room-temperature water with the juice of ½ of an organic lemon.

First meal of the day: 16 ounces of Tonijean's Raw Detox Juice. All organic ingredients are a must for optimal flavor, toxin-free consumption, and highest nutritional value.

> Through a juicer, press:
> 2 cucumbers with skin
> 1 green lime with skin
> 2 large carrots with or without the leaves
> 1 green apple with skin
> 4–6 leaves of fresh dandelion
> 4–6 leaves of fresh romaine
> 6 stalks of fresh celery
>
> Once juice is pressed, add ½ teaspoon of organic spirulina powder to your juice and shake in the powder well.

This juice should be consumed within fifteen minutes. After thirty minutes, enjoy 2 cups of organic cubed watermelon and 1 cup of fresh blueberries.

Throughout the entire cleanse, you will drink eight to ten 8 ounce glasses of water infused with fresh produce throughout the day.

To make infused water, begin with 8–10 ounces of water. Some suggestions for products to add to water:

3 cucumber slices with skin and 2–3 small slices of apple with skin

OR add a few leaves of fresh mint or basil to the produce listed above

Alternate: add 2–3 pieces of orange with fresh mint or basil

Be creative with your infusions and add the produce you choose. Since produce is high in enzymes and antioxidants necessary for cleansing, you can have fun.

Lunch will consist of a delicious mixed green salad. Here's an example:

In your favorite salad bowl combine:
2 cups of either chopped, fresh romaine, kale, or arugula, or all three
4–5 cherry tomatoes
½ diced zucchini with skin
½ avocado, diced
3 strawberries, diced
½ yellow, orange, or red bell pepper cleaned and diced
¼ cup diced red onion
½ teaspoon garlic and onion powder mixed
Celtic or unrefined salt and black pepper to taste
2 forkfuls of alfalfa or broccoli sprouts
1 teaspooon raw chia seeds
1 tablespoon extra virgin olive oil mixed with ½ teaspoon raw hempseed oil
1 teaspoon raw apple cider or coconut vinegar

Toss with love and enjoy!

Midafternoon blender snack:

> 8 ounces of raw coconut water
> 1 tablespoon raw coconut oil
> 1 small or medium banana ripe
> ¾ to 1 cup frozen or fresh mixed organic berries
> 1 teaspoons raw hempseeds
> ½ teaspoon organic vanilla extract
> ½ tablespoon raw bee pollen granules

Blend with love and enjoy!

Dinner: Enjoy a meal of vegetables, protein, and healthy fat.

> You may have any green vegetable of your choice: steamed broccoli, kale, spinach, brussel sprouts, or green cabbage.

> If you eat meat, you may have: grass-fed beef, wild fish, or pastured chicken or eggs.

> If you do not eat meat, you may have ½–1 cup organic beans of your choice seasoned with garlic, onion, fresh herbs, real salt, and black pepper.

> Add two or more forkfuls of raw, lacto-fermented sauerkraut to your plate for healthy digestion.

> You may include a baked or boiled sweet potato or 2 ounces of organic, pre-soaked, germinated quinoa or brown rice.

> You may add organic butter or ghee.

> Seasoning your food with real salt is perfectly fine, as these minerals are critical.

You will need to follow this meal plan exactly as stated for all three days during the detox, and no other food sources are allowed during the three days. Please be sure to consume your water infusions throughout the day.

Tonijean's Gentle Detox Bath

Your skin is your largest organ, as well as your external immune system. In the evening before bed, you must take a detox bath.

1. Fill your tub with hot water that is comfortable for you, adding 1 cup of Epsom salt or Dead Sea salt.

2. Add a few drops of each: peppermint, chamomile, lemon, and lavender essential oils to your bath water.

3. While the water is filling up, dry brush for 5-7 minutes to stimulate your immune and lymphatic systems and expel toxins.

4. Relax in the bath for 15–20 minutes.

5. After the bath, massage chamomile oil to the bottoms of your feet— approximately 3-4 drops to each foot.

Congratulate yourself; you have completed your first day of Tonijean's Simple Cleanse. Don't be alarmed if you see parasites in your bath water, as this is a successfully sign of cleansing— these could be external parasites, such as scabies or lice, or internal parasites, such as pinworms.

This bath will be repeated for all three days to complete the detox.

Coffee Enemas

You may enhance the cleansing process by having coffee enemas. Coffee enemas are extremely beneficial for the removal of dangerous parasites in the intestines and colon.

A coffee enema is an insertion of organic coffee via the anus to cleanse the rectum, colon, and large intestines of harmful toxins. The mucosa lining in our colon nests many different species of parasites that eventually result in disease. Coffee enemas safely rid the body of constipation, candida, and parasites. This procedure is necessary for healing the body of various health conditions.

Why Coffee?

You're probably wondering why coffee is used to clean out toxins from our colon. Coffee is a high-antioxidant plant that has a large role in herbal medicine. Coffee has potent properties for liver cleansing—and most people today have a toxic liver. The high level of antioxidants found in coffee flush heavy metals, fungi, and toxins out of the colon. Every day we are exposed to chemicals from the air we breathe, the water we drink, and the foods we eat.

Caffeinated coffee is preferred. The caffeine is preferentially absorbed into the system and goes directly to the liver, where it then becomes a strong detoxicant. It causes the liver to produce more bile-containing processed toxics and moves bile out toward the small intestine for elimination.

A Simple Coffee Enema

Purchase a standard enema bag. These can be ordered online or found at a local drugstore or pharmacy.

Preparing the coffee: Add three flat tablespoons of ground organic, caffeinated coffee to 2 quarts of distilled or pure spring water. Add heat. Allow the coffee to come to a boil for three minutes, then simmer for approximately twenty minutes. Strain the grains from the coffee using a cheesecloth and cool until the liquid is a comfortable temperature. Make sure the coffee is lukewarm or body temperature, not hot.

Hang your enema bag close in a warm area near a toilet. Lubricate the end of the enema tube with coconut oil or Vaseline. Relax and lie on your left side and gently insert the tube into your rectum with your knees pulled up close to your chest. Anatomical positioning of the lower colon will help the fluid go directly into the colon. Using the enema bag, gently release the clamp so the fluid will flow into your colon.

While lightly massaging your abdomen, try and hold the liquid for at least three minutes, depending on your ability to tolerate the pressure in the abdominal area. As your colon is filling with the liquid, a normal feeling of fullness will occur. The ability to hold the liquid for longer times improves with practice. The longer the liquid is held, the greater the removal of poisons from the colon and liver. Do not force yourself to hold more liquid than you can handle when you begin this practice. This will become easier over time as you perform more enemas.

Eliminate the liquid and fecal matter by expelling into the toilet and repeat the procedure one or more times until all the liquid in the enema bag has been used. It is extremely common to feel some discomfort during or after an enema, which may include cramping, nausea, or light-headedness. These are all normal signs that your body is ridding itself of toxins. You may resume normal eating after an enema, but avoid non-organic and processed foods.

For additional information on coffee enemas, please refer to the book *Wellness Against All Odds*, by Dr. Sherry Rogers (Prestige Publishing, 1994).

Please consult your medical doctor or a qualified physician before beginning any type of cleansing or detox procedure, including enemas.

Laughter Is Medicine

There's nothing like a good belly laugh. Laughter brings people together and boosts immune cells called *killer T cells*. Laughter increases infection-fighting antibodies, improving your resistance to disease. Laughing stimulates serotonin in the brain, decreases stress hormones, and releases endorphins, the body's natural feel-good chemicals. Endorphins promote an overall sense of well-being and can even temporarily relieve pain.

> *A cheerful heart is good medicine, but a crushed spirit dries up the bones.*
>
> — Proverbs 17:22 NIV

Yoga

Yoga is a practical aid, not a religion. It soothes the soul while toning the body. Yoga is a practice contained in Hindu spiritual and ascetic disciplines. People have been practicing this healing modality for well more than five thousand years. The word *yoga* comes from Sanskrit, an ancient Indian language, which means to integrate or unite.

Performing yoga encourages harmonizing the body through various breathing techniques, simple meditation, and specific bodily postures. Many practitioners, including myself, have recommend yoga as a part of a successful healing protocol. Patients have experienced relief from chronic illnesses, as well as healthy behavioral changes. Yoga is widely practiced around the world for health and relaxation. Practicing yoga helps eliminate negative interferences that block our subconscious perception from truth.

No matter what ails your aching body, yoga is right for anyone. Here are some of the many health benefits of practicing yoga:

- Cardio and circulatory improvement
- Improved athletic performance
- Increased energy and vitality
- Weight reduction
- Increased strength and endurance
- Improved flexibility
- Toned muscles

Yoga can also lower blood pressure and reduce insomnia. I highly suggest that yoga becomes part of your healing regimen.

Rest and Sleep Are NOT a Luxury

Proper rest and sleep are critical for health. Most people today avoid taking time to rest properly and sleep enough. Everyone seems to be in a rush, running here and there while rest is last on the list. Taking time for ourselves is important to release stress and build wellness in the body. Proper rest and adequate sleep help us better manage stress.

Sleep is often the missing component in health, and without a good night's sleep, we feel short-circuited.

Have you ever experienced a headache or belly ache from a lack of sleep? Sleep makes you feel better, but its benefits go far beyond getting rid of those dark circles and a belly ache.

A lack of sleep can cause digestive issues, headaches, constipation, fatigue, mood swings, and even weight gain. You require proper rest and sleep to maintain hormonal balance. Hormonal imbalances contribute to thyroid issues and extra pounds. Sleep deprivation may also cause loss of concentration, memory issues, and a lack of motivation. Prolonged sleep issues over time contribute to heart issues, diabetes, and a compromised immune system that could lead to cancer.

A good night's rest allows the body to detox and heal. The liver rejuvenates between the hours of 10:00 p.m. and 2:00 a.m., and the kidneys go into a state of dialysis. Sleeping at the correct hours is important for optimal organ function. You can catch up on lost sleep from a few days. However, if you continue to have poor sleep patterns, it is difficult for your body to restore its rest. Every hour that you sleep before midnight adds to your health while every hour of sleep that you lose after 10:30 p.m. robs from your health.

I'm a dreamer; every night I dream. Sometimes my dreams are a bit strange and other times my dreams are interesting. I seem to enjoy talking about my dreams when I wake.

Dreaming is important; it indicates that our bodies went into deeper sleep called the *Rapid Eye Movement* (REM) sleep cycle. There are three phases of non-REM sleep. Each stage can last from five to fifteen minutes. You must go through all three phases to reach REM sleep. The first sleep cycle each night contains relatively short periods of REM, and you can easily be awakened during this phase. Longer periods of deep sleep happen as the night progresses. Periods of REM sleep increase in length during the deeper sleep cycles. The REM cycle takes 90 to 110 minutes after you've fallen asleep.

Sleep deprivation symptoms include having a difficult time getting out of bed in the morning and a feeling of sluggishness in the afternoon. One may also experience sleepiness during the day and a need to nap to get through the rest of the day. Other symptoms may include falling asleep while watching television or falling asleep within five minutes of going to bed.

A feeling of irritability and mood swings are also common with sleep-deprived individuals.

There may be a difference between the amount of sleep you get and the amount of sleep that you need. Even if you're able to operate on a few hours of sleep each night, that doesn't mean your body doesn't require more. You may be surprised, but you'll feel a lot better and accomplish more if you spend an extra hour or two in bed. Trading away sleep for other *important* things may cause you harm.

Check out the chart below to see how much sleep is required for humans at different ages.

> Newborn–12 months: 12–18 hours of sleep
> 3 months–1 year: 14 hours of sleep
> 1–3 years: 12–14 hours of sleep
> 3–5 years: 11–13 hours of sleep
> 5–12 years: 10–11 hours of sleep
> 12–18 years: 8 ½–10 hours of sleep
> 18 years +: 7 ½–9 hours of sleep

Sleep Naked

Forget your pajamas and reap the benefits of sleeping naked. According to The National Sleep Foundation, sleeping in your birthday suit will actually lead to better, deeper sleep without the distractions of clothing. Removing your clothing before bed also regulates hormones, such as melatonin and cortisol, keeping your endocrine system in balance. When you sleep naked, it helps your body temperature naturally regulate cortisol, the stress hormone, keeping your levels in an optimal range. Lower stress levels can also reduce your blood pressure levels.

Wearing multiple layers of clothing all day doesn't allow your armpits, feet, and private parts a chance to breathe. This factor can raise your risk of infections, athlete's foot, and skin diseases. If you're married or living with a significant other, sleeping naked may also energize your sex life, increasing skin-to-skin contact.

Ditching the PJs also releases the feel-good hormones oxytocin, serotonin, and dopamine, which are your love neurotransmitters. A good night's rest increases great health, enhances mood, and creates a healthy glow. If you are feeling ill or just too cold, then clothing may be necessary to prevent further illness and discomfort. Sleeping naked is a step in the right direction to better health. So, go commando!

Prayer

Prayer is a two-way communication between you and God. Prayer allows you to speak with God and hear His voice. The solemn request of prayer also allows you to express your love and thankfulness to God as a form of worship. The closeness of praying invites assurance, peace, calmness, and security from our Almighty God.

Anger and Un-forgiveness

It's obvious that I believe in the importance of healthy, organic, whole foods, healing modalities, and proper rest and sleep. I also want to emphasize the importance of forgiveness. Carrying anger and un-forgiveness is like drinking poison and expecting the other person to die. Anger and un-forgiveness harbor sickness and disease inside our bodies no matter what we eat or drink. Please forgive those that have wronged you, as God has forgiven you.

> *For if you forgive others their trespasses, your heavenly Father will also forgive you, but if you do not forgive others their trespasses, neither will your Father forgive your trespasses.*
>
> — Matthew 6:14 ESV

CHAPTER SEVENTEEN

Coffee and Tea

Many people ask if they should remove coffee from their diet; you might be surprised with my answer. I believe from my extensive research that coffee is a healthy beverage, full of antioxidants known to prevent disease. Keep in mind that non-organic coffee can be an unhealthy beverage. Non-organic coffee is a chemically treated beverage. It is steeped in synthetic fertilizers, pesticides, herbicides, fungicides, and insecticides. You must follow these two principles to make coffee a health food and not an unhealthy habit.

Here are the pros and cons of what's in your cup.

Coffee

Coffee should be organic, making it optimally nutritious. Coffee that's not organic is full of disease-forming compounds that result in sickness. Conventional coffee is high in pesticides and other chemical fertilizers. Organic coffee can be a healthy choice for a hot or iced beverage.

We should not rely on coffee for our energy. Overconsumption of caffeine can become addictive, and thus an unhealthy choice.

Coffee drinkers, if you consume more than two six ounce cups per day, cutting back on your intake is a wise idea. Non-coffee drinkers, there's no need to *start* drinking coffee, as there are other sources of beneficial antioxidants.

Coffee is a potent source of healthy antioxidants. In fact, coffee has as many antioxidants as green tea and raw cacao, two high antioxidant-rich foods. Coffee has high ORAC levels. ORAC is *oxygen radical absorbance capacity* or antioxidant capacity. Antioxidants are substances that inhibit oxidation that causes internal damage that eventually results in disease. There are one thousand antioxidants in unprocessed coffee beans and hundreds more develop during the roasting process.

I can almost smell the fresh-brewed aroma; can you?

Antioxidants fight inflammation, an underlying cause of many chronic conditions, such as autoimmune conditions, arthritis, atherosclerosis, and many types of cancer. Antioxidants neutralize free radicals, which cause oxidative stress and accelerate aging. Free radicals lead to poor cellular function and chronic disease. Antioxidants are critical in helping us stay healthy by protecting our cells from free radical damage.

Do you understand how important antioxidants are by this point?

Chlorogenic acid, an antioxidant found in coffee, also helps prevent cardiovascular disease, reduces the risk of kidney stones, boosts memory, lowers depression, and curbs cancer risk.

Polyphenols, antioxidant phytochemicals found in coffee, are recognized as anti-carcinogenic in studies and help reduce inflammation responsible for some tumors (Jong, 2014). To obtain optimal nutritional value in your coffee, your choice should be organic to receive the benefits as well as avoiding the damaging health effects of chemical fertilizers. Now that you've learned coffee is a nutritious beverage, let's talk about some cons of drinking coffee.

Coffee drinkers, I know you're happy to learn that drinking coffee has health benefits, but more is not necessarily better. In some cases, coffee causes irritability, nervousness, or anxiety in higher quantities, and it can impact sleep patterns, causing insomnia. Coffee consumption can raise blood pressure, which should be a consideration for people with high blood pressure. Thankfully, the elevation in blood pressure is temporary— no longer than several hours— and research indicates that there is no correlation between coffee drinking and long-term incidences in elevated blood pressure (Jong, 2014).

Caffeine Caution

Caffeine affects every person differently. Consider cutting back on your coffee drinking if you suffer side effects. It takes about six hours for the effects of caffeine to wear off, so drink coffee early in the day. Another option is to switch to organic decaf, which contains about 2-12 mg of caffeine per eight ounces. If you want to limit your coffee consumption, wean down your coffee consumption gradually. Quitting abruptly can lead to uncomfortable caffeine withdrawal symptoms. These symptoms may include severe headache, insomnia, muscle and joint pain, lack of concentration, and sleepiness.

What is a healthy amount of coffee? Moderate coffee drinkers have two or three cups (8 ounces) per day. Heavy coffee drinkers have four cups or more. The amount of caffeine per coffee beverage varies; eight ounces of regular brewed coffee may contain as little as 80 to as much as 200 mg of caffeine per cup (Jong, 2014).

The bottom line: if you are sensitive to caffeine, please use coffee with caution. Drinking non-organic coffee can put poison in your cup, so be sure you choose organic. Limiting your daily intake to 1-2 cups is wise. I believe that your energy should be obtained from a good quality night's sleep and good sources of nutrition. No, America should not run on coffee.

Tea

Tea is a miraculous healing beverage loaded with antioxidants and health benefits. Herbal tea has high antioxidant properties and energy-boosting effects. Tea is also calming, soothing, and relaxing.

Tea, as well as all drinks and foods, should be organic to avoid disease-forming compounds found in chemical fertilizers. Tea can be enjoyed over ice in the summer or steaming hot in the winter. A beverage for all seasons, tea boosts your health while generating serenity and comfort.

What could be lurking in this naturally healing beverage? Let's examine the harmful chemicals that could be soaking in your teacup. If you have been drinking conventional herbal teas thinking they are a healthy choice, I have some upsetting news.

Most conventional teas contain chemical fertilizers and genetically modified ingredients. Conventional teas also have added artificial ingredients, including *fake* flavors and colors. The marketing for these teas contain words, such as *no artificial colors*, yet the ingredients list says *all natural flavorings*. Don't be fooled! The word *flavorings* is an indication that the ingredients are artificial. The added flavors in these tea sources contain a host of chemicals, such as crude oil and coal tar and are topped with a deceiving label stating that the product is *all natural*. The deception doesn't stop there.

Consider tea packaging. The little mesh and silky sachets that carry the leaves for your hot or cold beverages are loaded with a laundry list of harsh poisons. Some dangerous packagings include lead, nylon, or *polyethylene terephthalate*, and plastics, such as *polylactic acid* or PLA. These substances are known as cancer-causing agents. Paper tea bags also contain plenty of disease-forming elements. They contain highly carcinogenic compounds, such as *epichlorohydrin*, a strong irritant and carcinogen. Now that's a mouthful. The National Institute for Occupational Safety and Health (cdc.gov/niosh) claims these toxoids have the potential to cause infertility, impaired immune function, and cancer.

Please be aware of these highly chemical-laden brands that you may have trusted as your source of tea for yourself and your family:

- Celestial Seasonings
- Twinnings
- Teavanna
- Wellness Tea
- Tazo
- Bigelow
- Lipton
- Tea Forte
- Trader Joe's

These brands have shown high levels of cancer-causing toxins, with some as high as twenty-three different pesticides, herbicides and, insecticides. These chemical cocktails are highly carcinogenic pesticides that soak into your steaming hot tea water.

Don't be deceived by loose-leaf, high-end tea brands, as these have also tested positive for dangerous pesticides. Just because these teas are without the packaging doesn't mean they are any better. Look for organic loose leaf tea. Some reputable brands I recommend are California Tea House, Upton Tea Exports, and Frontier Coop organic tea.

A Final Word

Be aware that if a product says *all natural*, it does not mean that the product has any true quality, chemical free, or organic. These words indicate that ingredients came from nature at one time. Although some brands may appear high quality and natural, they may have pesticide-ridden packaging. There are many deceiving brands of teas and coffees out there with tempting labels. They mislead you with marketing. You must make organic, non-GMO your only choice. Remember, herbal teas and coffees are healthy beverages, but your health relies on the source that you choose. Purchasing organic teas and coffee will assure you that you're buying non-GMO, chemical and pesticide free — including healthy packaging.

Coffee and tea can be nutritious and comforting, whether hot or cold. Please allow these guidelines to assist you when shopping for tea and coffee, so these beverages will benefit your health.

Sources of coffee and herbal teas can be found in the resources section of this book.

CHAPTER EIGHTEEN

Water, the Basis of All Life Force

Whoever believes in me . . . rivers of living water will flow from within them.

—John 7:38 NIV

Throughout this book you have learned the importance of real, whole, organic foods and their many health benefits. However, to benefit from the nutrients in your food effectively, you must drink enough water. Water is an odorless, tasteless liquid that fills the oceans, rivers, and seas, from rain. Water is a living substance and is necessary for the health of all life forms.

Water has a two-part delivery system: transport and export. Water transports nutrients from our food into our cells and exports toxins from our tissues, cells, and organs out of our bodies.

Many years ago, no one thought that we would live in such a polluted world that we would no longer be able to drink water from the tap or need to purchase safe drinking water through filtering systems and bottling. Now, we find ourselves trying to figure out what type of water is best for our consumption and where to find it. Who would have ever thought that one day we would need to purchase water?

This chapter will deliver a breakdown of the different types of water, including their pros and cons.

Natural Drinking Water

Water in its purest form includes spring water, snow, ice, rain, morning dew, and live coconut water. These are all forms of H_2O, hydrogen and oxygen. Real, live water that is beneficial to humans, animals, and plants is water that is free of contaminants. These contaminants include fluoride, chloride, copper, and other metals. These contaminants may be leaking from your pipes and are neurotoxic to the brain and other organs.

Staying hydrated is a key component, or the missing link, leading to optimal health. Symptoms of dehydration can be minor or severe and are as follows:

- Headaches
- Excessive hunger
- Skin problems
- Digestive issues
- Nutritional deficiencies
- Insomnia
- Autointoxication or self-poisoning
- Heart disease
- Cancer

Tap water from municipal water systems is considered *dead* water since all its life force has been destroyed and harsh pollutants have been added. Dead water is like processed foods, altered from their origin through pasteurization and other chemical processing.

Well water pumped up from under the ground may contain high levels of pesticides, nitrates, pharmaceutical residues, radon, and lead. I suggest you have your water tested regularly by a reputable water company.

If your tap water is *hard,* then it likely contains lime scale, a dangerous form of calcium that is not safe for human consumption and contributes to many health issues. Once its beneficial bacteria are lost through high processing, this dead water is no longer beneficial to us. Tap water is obviously not a wise choice for drinking water.

Real spring water is extremely beneficial to us and therefore is the best type of water for optimal oxygen delivery.

What are some of the other sources of water?

Distilled Water

Distilled water is created through the process of distillation. Pure H_2O is boiled, releasing its contaminants. Many of the contaminants found in water are inorganic compounds, such as metals and minerals. This type of water is considered steam-cleaned water since all its impurities are gone.

Distilled water is not a wise choice, because the loss of electrolytes and trace minerals like magnesium can create deficiencies in the body, contributing to heartbeat irregularities and high blood pressure. Cooking in distilled water isn't any better. Distilled water pulls the minerals out of the foods to replace its own mineral loss and destroys the foods' nutritional value.

Distilled water is an active absorber of carbon dioxide: an odorless, tasteless, colorless gas, making distilled water highly acidic. When one consumes distilled water in larger quantities, it creates an acidic gut environment, which makes one more susceptible to disease. Distilled water should be used only in small quantities and infrequently.

Purified or Filtered Water

Purified water is any type of water that has been cleansed and purified through mechanically filtered processes to remove chemicals or contaminants. These processes include reverse osmosis, distillation, or deionization. There is little difference between purified, filtered, and distilled water except purified water goes through other processes called reverse osmosis, *ozonation*, ion exchange, and sand filtration.

Ozonation is a chemical water treatment technique that disinfects against bacteria in the water. If you do not have any other water source, then purified or filtered water is better than not drinking any water at all.

Bottled Water

Most bottled waters are purified or spring water. Both are fine when you're thirsty, as hydration is important. Spring water is a better option than purified since it's closer to what nature provides. Plastic bottles are the main concern. We need to be aware that each year about two million tons of plastic bottles end up in landfills in the United States alone. This means more waste, less oil, and more costs for the environment, wildlife, and humanity.

Plastic isn't just bad for the planet; it's not good for you and me. There are many chemicals in most bottled water on the market today. We need to be aware.

Bottled Water Quality

High quality environmental laboratories found thirty-eight contaminants in ten brands of bottled water purchased from grocery stores — including Wal-Mart — in several states around the country (Naidenko, 2008). The pollutants identified include disinfection byproducts, chemical fertilizer residue, and waste-water pollutants from pharmaceuticals. Some of these contaminants contained an array of cancer-causing byproducts from municipal tap water. These elements include chlorination, heavy metals and minerals, arsenic, radioactive isotopes, and chemical fertilizers.

Reverse Osmosis

Reverse osmosis is one process by which water is processed and *purified*. Water under pressure moves through a semipermeable membrane to demineralize or deionize water and remove the larger contaminants.

Reverse osmosis dissolves inorganic solids, such as salts, which are then removed from the water solution. One disadvantage of reverse osmosis water is the water is demineralized. The semi-permeable membrane used in the process removes any beneficial mineral particles, including sodium, calcium, magnesium, and iron since they are larger than water molecules.

Reverse osmosis does have certain benefits, considering there are ways to bypass some of its disadvantages. Unlike most carbon filter systems, reverse osmosis will remove the fluoride that most municipalities in the United States add to their water. This process removes most contaminants from the water, especially when combined with a pre- and post-carbon filtration system. If your water source is fluoridated, reverse osmosis will successfully remove this neurotoxin from your water.

Fluoride is more poisonous than lead and slightly less poisonous than arsenic. Fluoride is a cumulative poison that accumulates in bone over the years. Consumption of a little bit of this poison every day in your drinking water and shower can lead to *osteosarcoma*, known as bone cancer. Osteosarcoma has been reported in areas that have higher levels of fluoride in the water. This neurological toxin also causes thyroid and endocrine conditions, lower IQ levels, and memory and concentration issues.

Fluoride has the potential to cause skin eruptions, such as atopic dermatitis, eczema, or urticarial. It can also cause gastric distress, headache, and weakness in muscles. Avoiding fluoride treatments at your next dentist visit is a wise choice, as this treatment has been known to cause *fluorosis* of the teeth. Fluorosis is hypomineralization of the tooth enamel caused by the ingestion of excessive fluoride. Fluorosis appears as brown spots or discoloration on your teeth after several fluoride treatments.

Fluoride was dumped into our water supply as a cheap means of disposal of this toxic waste. The public was told that fluoride was good for teeth. This misconception was an evil yet easier method of distribution than paying the price to get rid of toxic fluoride safely. Ingesting this toxic poison is no different than swallowing toxic hair color or clothes detergent. As it is a liquid, fluoride will travel rapidly into the bloodstream.

Chlorine is a toxic gas that is used for sanitation, sewage, and industrial waste, yet it's added to swimming pools and drinking water.

Chlorine and fluoride are not the only dangers in drinking tap water. There are estrogen-mimicking hormones, herbicides, pesticides, drug residues, as well as heavy metals. These elements all keep us at risk of developing a laundry list of health conditions, starting with:

- Wheezing
- Asthma
- Allergies
- Digestive issues
- Hormonal imbalances
- Blood disorders
- Autointoxication or self-poisoning
- Brain and neurological issues
- Stomach, kidney, and bladder cancers

Alkaline Water

Alkaline water has recently become popular, but I am not a fan of this current craze. Most alkaline waters on the market are artificially alkaline and can cause many health issues.

Water in general is mostly neutral—not acidic or too alkaline. Natural alkaline water is generally considered safe since it contains natural minerals. However, you should avoid artificial alkaline water, which probably contains fewer minerals than you require for good health. Overuse of this water could leave you mineral-deficient.

Water that is naturally alkaline occurs when water passes over rocks and picks up minerals that increase its alkaline level. This water is quite safe. Your body cannot become too alkaline or acidic with natural alkaline water because your body recognizes this water and knows what to do. Artificial alkaline waters can make you highly acidic. The high artificial alkalinity content makes your body start pumping out levels of hydrochloric acid; many people then become highly acidic.

This water may produce good results for the first month; however, don't be fooled. There will eventually be many side effects, creating serious complications. The human body must be alkaline and acid balanced; being too alkaline or too acidic has the potential to kill off normal healthy cells.

The danger in alkaline water is that it is artificially transformed into alkaline water by a process called *ionizing*. The process of ionizing is an artificial process. Ionizing water or water *electrolysis* is a process that increases the alkalinity in water by adding minerals to the water. Like food that has been genetically altered, it is no longer recognized by the body. If your alkaline water is not naturally occurring, then you need to avoid it at all costs.

Seltzer or Carbonated Water

Seltzer is not the best choice for your digestion. Carbonated water creates too much gas in your digestive system, leading to flatulence and burping. It may irritate or initiate ulcers. If you already have digestive issues, carbonated water may cause bloating and abdominal discomfort.

Heartburn or reflux occurs when the sphincter in the esophagus allows the contents of your stomach to regurgitate back up into your esophagus. Carbonated drinks disrupt digestion, making these symptoms even worse. Some carbonated waters also contain artificial flavorings, such as lemon or lime, which may increase acidic content, making heartburn worse.

One of my remedies for heartburn is:

> Start with 6–8 ounces of warm water, not hot water. Add 1 tablespoon of raw apple cider vinegar and sip over a

period of three to four minutes until liquid is completely gone.

This is a miracle heartburn reliever without the health effects of prescription drugs or over-the-counter heartburn medication.

Headaches, body aches, mood swings, gut issues, excessive hunger, and dry skin.

Does this sound like you?

You may very well be dehydrated! Be sure to hydrate your cells daily no matter the season. Your body always needs water.

Most headaches can be relieved by drinking 8–10 ounces of water, waiting ten minutes and drinking another glass of water before reaching for aspirin. About 75 percent of Americans suffer from dehydration.

My best suggestion for your optimal water source is go online to findaspring.com for a local spring water source in your area and fill up your glass or steel bottles. I also suggest professional water filters and systems, as well as excellent bottled water companies.

My top suggestions include:

Healthy Perception water purification systems
healthyperceptions.com

New Wave Enviro Products
newwaveenviro.com

Dr. Mercola's water filtration systems
waterfilters.mercola.com

Reign water by Beyond Organic
healthfoodemporium.com/beyond-organic

Evamor water
evamor.com

Fiji water
fijiwater.com

How Much Water Is Enough?

I am often asked how much water a person should be drinking. The answer to that question depends on your weight. One should consume half an ounce of water for every pound that you weigh. In other words, if you weigh 150 pounds, then you need to drink seventy-five ounces daily. This amount is equal to half your weight in water.

A healthy bladder can hold one-and-a-half to two cups of water during the daytime and about four cups during sleep. It is normal to pass urine six or seven times a day if you are consuming six to eight glasses of water.

Fruit-Infused Water

Infused water has cut up, fresh organic fruits, herbs, or veggies added to pure water. Infused water relieves dehydration, delivers instant energy, creates radiant, glowing skin and is a wonderful refreshing alternative to the chemical-laden soft drinks on the market.

Be creative and make your own recipes by adding your favorite fresh herbs, veggies, and fruits to a half or whole gallon of water, storing overnight for best results. You may double your ingredients for larger quantities.

Here are some recipes for infused water that I love to drink, especially on a hot summer day. I suggest organic ingredients for optimal flavor and highest nutritional value.

Recipe # 1

>2 fresh mint leaves
>3-4 slices of fresh cucumber with skin
>1 sliced fresh lemon or lime with skin
>Add to 16-32 ounces of pure water

Recipe # 2

>2 strawberries, chopped
>3-4 blueberries, whole
>3-4 raspberries, whole
>3-4 grapes
>Add to 16-32 ounces of pure water

Recipe # 3

>½ organic apple, chopped with skin
>3 orange slices
>1 handful of fresh cranberries
>1 sprig of fresh rosemary
>Add to 16-32 ounces of pure water

CHAPTER NINETEEN

I Want to Spice Up Your Life

Definitions

Spice is the term used to describe parts of plants that are used to enhance the flavor or color of food. Spices can be seeds, fruits, berries, bark, buds, roots, or vegetable.

Essential oils are concentrations of original oils. Essential oils have features of the plant, such as flavor and aroma. Essential oils increase our sense of well-being, wholeness, and our connection to healing from within.

An *extract* is a derivative of highly concentrated aromatic oils from a plant.

> *And they cast out many demons, and anointed with oil many who were sick, and healed them.*
> — Mark 6:13 ESV

Spices and essential oils have been around since ancient biblical times. They have been used as medicine successfully for the prevention of diseases. They have also been used for cosmetic purposes and for their spiritual and emotional attributes. Spices were also used for pickling or seasonings to add flavor, vitamins, and minerals to hearty meals. Spices are not used as the main ingredient in foods and cosmetics due to their intense flavor and color.

Herbs, spices, and essential oils have made a huge comeback today for their *roborant*—strengthening—properties. I incorporate many spices as often as needed and desired for the medicinal benefits and abundant flavors. I suggest you do the same.

> *I have sprinkled my bed with myrrh, aloes, and cinnamon. Come, let us drink our fill of love until morning; Let us delight ourselves with caresses.*
> —Proverbs 7:17 NAS

Cinnamon

Cinnamon is a spice that is made from the inner bark of an evergreen tree, *Cinnamomum*. It is one of my favorite spices. I love it so much, I use it every day in a smoothie. Cinnamon is one of the most delicious and healthiest spices on the planet.

Cinnamon is a natural anti-inflammatory. It is beneficial in the reduction of arthritis, rheumatism, heart attack risk, blood pressure, and lowering blood sugar levels. Cinnamon helps improve the glycemic status, including levels of fasting blood glucose, among people with type 2 diabetes. Cinnamon improves your body's ability to regulate blood glucose levels.

This incredible spice has been used as a medicinal ingredient throughout history, dating back as far as ancient Egypt. Cinnamon used to be rare and valuable, regarded as a gift fit for kings. In ancient and biblical times, cinnamon was once considered more precious than gold, and has some amazing medicinal benefits. The bark was traditionally collected for anointing oil as well as perfume.

Today cinnamon has become one of the most popular spices in the holistic industry. Cassia cinnamon is the most commonly used variety; however, Ceylon cinnamon is best.

Choosing the right cinnamon makes all the difference. The most common cinnamon available in supermarkets today is not real cinnamon at all. You must look for Ceylon, which is known as the *true* cinnamon. Usually Ceylon cinnamon is labeled, so if you have unlabeled, whole cinnamon sticks, these are from the plant bark of cassia.

Ceylon cinnamon bark will be thinner with more layers, compared to the thicker bark of cassia. Ceylon cinnamon has higher levels of medicinal properties.

The sweet, delicate spice of Ceylon is preferred over cassia by many dessert lovers, including myself. Both types of cinnamon carry similar health benefits, but take note that cassia cinnamon should only be used in small quantities. Cassia contains a natural plant chemical called *coumarin* that acts as a blood thinner. This chemical is contraindicated for anyone taking prescription blood thinners. The coumarin present in cassia cinnamon can be toxic to the liver and kidneys, which may negate any of its benefits.

Ceylon cinnamon contains antioxidant compounds called *proanthocyanadins*. These resemble the antioxidant compounds found in green tea, berries, and grapes. Coumarin-free Ceylon cinnamon may also be beneficial to the liver, according to studies reviewed by *BMC Complementary and Alternative*

Medicine in 2013, with no adverse effects to other organ systems (Ranasinghe, 2013).

Proanthocyanadins are condensed tannins, or naturally occurring antioxidants. They play a critical role in the metabolic processes in the body. The antioxidant power in proanthocyanadins is 20 percent higher than vitamin C and 50 percent higher than vitamin E, two critical immune-boosting nutrients. These compounds have been shown to promote healthy skin and cell health due to their ability to bond with *collagen*, a necessary protein found in connective tissues.

Other benefits of Ceylon cinnamon include antimicrobial and antiparasitic activity, which benefit digestive health. Cinnamon may be the solution for diabetes, Candida, weight loss, cancer, Alzheimer's, arthritis, Parkinson's, anxiety, and much more.

> There's good reason to use cinnamon for more than a boost to your morning beverage. Cinnamon enhances antioxidant defenses, and it kills E. coli and many other bacteria. Its anti-inflammatory compounds help relieve pain and stiffness of muscles and joints due to arthritis.
>
> Research published in the journal Molecular Biology states that chronic inflammation plays a major role in the development of various neurodegenerative diseases, including Alzheimer's disease, Parkinson's disease, multiple sclerosis, brain tumor, and meningitis. (Mercola, 2015)

Cassia

All your robes are fragrant with myrrh and aloes and cassia, from palaces adorned with ivory, the music of the strings makes you glad.

— Psalms 45:8 NIV

In biblical times, cassia oil was used for anointing. Cassia has aromatic properties that resemble cinnamon. Cassia is used today as a natural hair color and conditioner. The dried leaves are ground into a powder used for hair care products.

Cassia essential oil has medicinal use as an:

- Antidiarrheal
- Antidepressant
- Antimicrobial
- Antifungal
- Antirheumatic
- Antiarthritic
- Astringent
- Antiviral

Emotionally, Cassia essential oil encourages a person's sense of self-worth, inner strength, and courage. It may help support a person's confidence, increasing their willingness to try new things.

Add 1-2 drops of cassia oil to tea or coffee to promote healthy immune function, a warming and uplifting aroma, and healthy digestion.

Ginger

Ginger root is another favorite of mine. Ginger has a long history of relieving digestive problems, such as nausea, loss of appetite, and motion sickness. Ginger is a Southeast Asian herbacaceous perennial plant with an orange-brown color. Ginger is used chopped or powdered for cooking or juices, preserved as a syrup, or candied in sugar crystals.

Ginger also makes a wonderful cup of tea to soothe a sore throat or relieve an upset tummy. Try ginger in tea, soup, or capsules up to 250 milligrams four times a day. If you choose a carbonated beverage that contains ginger, check that it contains real ginger. The high anti-inflammatory properties in ginger make it a great pain reliever for the relief of headaches, menstrual cramps, and joint pain associated with arthritis. Ginger also contains antiviral, antibacterial, and antifungal properties. It ranks as one of the top antiparasitic herbs on the planet.

To combat motion sickness, take 1 gram of dried, powdered, encapsulated ginger thirty minutes to two hours before traveling. This spice can help ease travel-related nausea and motion sickness.

Nutmeg

Another wonderful way to spice up your health is with nutmeg. Its long list of health benefits includes:

- Relieves pain
- Soothes indigestion
- Strengthens cognitive function
- Detoxifies the body
- Boosts skin health
- Reduces insomnia

- Increases immune system function
- Reduces inflammation

Nutmeg acts as a natural detoxifier, removing toxins stored in the liver and kidneys. It helps dissolve kidney stones, increasing the overall function of the kidneys and liver.

Nutmeg is delicious in smoothies, desserts teas, or even savory dishes. It is another well-known spice that can be used for medicine as well as enhancing a recipe. You have another delicious, highly nutritious spice to add to your pantry.

Vanilla

Vanilla is like a dessert itself for its naturally sweet, candy-like flavor that adds just the right touch to almost any dessert. Vanilla is obtained from vanilla beans, which come from the orchids of the genus vanilla. This sweet, dark-colored extract is responsible for the delicious, popular vanilla ice cream that we all love as our favorite cold and creamy treat.

Be aware of products labeled vanilla *flavoring*. They are nothing but artificial, chemical versions of the real thing. There's absolutely nothing like real vanilla extract, and that is exactly what to buy.

Vanilla extract is not only richer tasting, but is packed with a wealth of nutritional benefits:

- Antioxidants
- Aphrodisiac
- Hormone balancing, regulates menstruation
- Tranquilizing and relaxing
- A natural antidepressant

Now, if you don't already have vanilla extract in your pantry, I will be shocked. I can only hope that you run out right now and purchase this wonderful extract.

Garlic

The famous garlic also known as *Allium sativum* is a strong, spicy, and pungent-tasting bulb that enhances the flavor of almost any dish. Garlic is a species of the onion genus, which includes shallots, rakkyo, chives, and leeks. Garlic is known for its medicinal purposes, typically as a natural antibiotic for treating colds and flus.

Garlic has been used as both food and medicine in many cultures for thousands of years, dating back to Egypt when the pyramids were built. Today, garlic is widely used to help prevent heart disease, including *atherosclerosis* or hardening of the arteries, a plaque buildup that can block the flow of oxygen and blood. This blockage may lead to a heart attack or stroke. Garlic also lowers blood pressure and purifies the blood. The enzymes in garlic have been found to be a potent weapon against cancer.

I love garlic and enjoy its aromatic flavor in most meals that I prepare, either cooked or raw. Garlic isn't only for keeping the vampires away. Garlic is successful in both powdered form and raw in its original form. Whether it's chopped, minced, powdered, or crushed — a little garlic goes a long way.

Oregano

Oregano is another herb known for its medicinal properties and is also used for cooking. Oregano belongs to the mint family. Its Latin name means *mountain joy*; it has a warm, aromatic, and balsamic flavor that is a perfect enhancement to most Mediterranean dishes.

I have successfully used oregano as medicine in my nutrition practice for patients suffering from:

- Colds
- Flus
- Respiratory conditions
- Menstrual cramps
- Urinary tract issues

Oregano adds just the right touch to hot or cold dishes. Use it fresh or dried.

Basil

Another super healing and delicious plant is basil, *Ocimum basilicum*, also known as Saint Joseph's Wort. This amazing herb also belongs to the mint family. Basil is known as the king of herbs or the *royal* herb and is native to India and other tropical areas of Asia.

I am definitely a fan of herbs and spices, and I am also in love with basil. Since I am of Italian decent, basil has been a long-time friend of mine in many dishes. Basil is not only wonderful in food, but it is also extremely high in anti-inflammatory agents. Basil contains two medicinal compounds called *orientin* and *vicenin*, two water-soluble flavonoids that have been known for their healing properties.

The basil plant's round, pointed leaves look a lot like its relative, peppermint. Basil is aromatic and sweet, yet has a peppery, anise flavor, which is why it is popular as the main ingredient in pesto. Both garlic and basil have brought the family to the dinner table many times in my home. The smell of fresh garlic and basil always reminds me of my grandmother, and although she has gone to be with the Lord, those wonderful aromas still bring me right back to her pesto.

You must try Grandma Frances's recipe for pesto. It was one of her specialties. Grandma would grind the basil by hand in an old-fashioned hand grinder. When my sister and I were kids, we used to ask grandma if she could make the green macaroni and she knew exactly what she needed to do.

Grandma Fran's Pesto

In a food processor or blender, add ingredients as follows:
1 large bunch of fresh basil leaves (about 2 cups, rinsed and dried)

3 medium cloves of fresh garlic

½ cup of raw pine nuts

¾ cup Parmesan, freshly grated (preferably imported sheep cheese for that traditional authentic Italian flavor)

Add 3–4 tablespoons of extra virgin olive oil to create a creamy, pourable, yet medium-thick consistency. Add a pinch of Celtic salt and a pinch of black pepper to taste.

I can almost smell it. Are you getting hungry? This typing is working up my appetite. I'd love to make this and have you come over and share it with me. My grandma would be proud.

Pesto is a raw dish, so all the nutrients and enzymes are active and ready for full nutrient delivery as you top this wonderful sauce on your favorite food. Pesto can be spread on top of sourdough bread or toast or as a dipping sauce for fresh veggies or sprouted, ancient grain pasta.

For a richer, creamier dish, we would add fresh raw cream from the farm, creating creamy pesto. Oh, my mouth is watering. How about yours?

Parsley

Parsley is a biennial plant with white flowers and either crinkly or flat leaves that are used as a culinary herb for flavor enhancement and garnishing. Parsley has a few flavors: salty, sour, bitter, and sweet or *umami*—meaning both sweet and sour—a loanword from the Japanese.

The herb parsley is more than a meal compliment or garnish. It is also used for its medicinal benefits.

Parsley:

- Supports the immune system with high antioxidant properties
- Assists in the body's ability to repair wounds quickly
- Stimulates bone health
- Flushes out excess fluid
- Supports healthy kidney function

I use a ton of parsley in my meals on a weekly basis for its wonderful health benefits and incredible flavor. I juice parsley as well as add it to soups, omelets, sautéed dishes, and salads.

Cilantro

Cilantro is another term for *coriander*, or Chinese parsley. Cilantro and parsley are similar in appearance, and I have a difficult time telling the difference. So, I smell it. Cilantro has a scent that can be compared to an insect, a stink bug. For some people, cilantro tastes like soap since soap and cilantro both contain *aldehyde*, a fruity green, pungent scent and taste. I love cilantro in salsa and soups for its unique flavor.

Cilantro is loaded with antioxidants, essential oils, vitamins, and dietary fiber. I use cilantro as a liver detoxifier for patients with liver health issues. It is beneficial in the prevention of liver problems, as well as in a healthy liver detox. Studies have shown that levels of heavy metals are purged from the body after drinking small amounts of freshly juiced cilantro.

For seasoning an Asian or Latin dish or a healthy detox, I highly suggest cilantro if you can get past the soapy taste and the scent of bugs.

Black Pepper

Black pepper is widely used as a spice and a condiment and may be used as whole peppercorns or ground. Black, green, and white pepper are technically fruit. Black pepper is used to preserve food as well as for flavoring and spicing up a dish. Black pepper is also known as a warming herb, which works well with turmeric and ginger, other warming herbs. Their potency is enhanced by using them together. Pepper is loaded with medicinal purposes, such as iron, manganese, potassium, vitamin K, vitamin C, and is a rich source of dietary fiber.

Cayenne Pepper

Let's heat things up a bit with America's red pepper.

Cayenne pepper is a strong, hot-tasting, red powder made from dried and ground red-hot chili peppers. Cayenne is more than a spice; it contains multiple medicinal health benefits. This pepper contains a natural pain reliever called *capsaicin*, which reduces headaches and joint pain.

Cayenne has anti-allergen properties, works as a digestive aide by stimulating intestinal peristaltic motion, supports healthy detox, and is a natural anti-inflammatory that helps control blood pressure. Cayenne peppers are related to jalapeños, and are a great spice to heat up chili as well as most meat and fish dishes. Cayenne is added to desserts by top culinary chefs.

Turmeric

Turmeric has a history of uses dating back four thousand years. Turmeric, or Indian saffron, is widely used in Indian dishes, stews, and chili. Turmeric is one of the most medicinal herbs on the planet, due to its anti-inflammatory properties.

Curcumin is the most important bio-active ingredient in turmeric, which contains high levels of antioxidants known to destroy cancer cells. Turmeric helps the body fight foreign invaders that contribute to disease. Studies have shown that turmeric has the potential to reverse the signs of oxidative damage that leads to Alzheimer's and other brain and neurological disorders.

Take a break from reading and start dinner with my vegetarian bean and turmeric chili that everyone will love.

Tonijean's Vegetarian Chili with Beans

Ingredients:

1 tablespoon virgin coconut oil
1 medium chopped onion
2 cloves minced garlic

½ red bell pepper, chopped

1½ teaspoon ground turmeric

2 teaspoons ground cumin

1 teaspoon ground onion powder

1 teaspoon ground garlic powder

Black pepper to taste

Celtic salt to taste

½ cup frozen or canned corn, drained

1 cup presoaked and cooked (or canned and drained) black beans

1 cup presoaked (or canned and drained) garbanzo beans, a.k.a. chick peas

1 cup presoaked (or canned and drained) red kidney beans

32 ounces crushed tomatoes

6–8 tablespoons whole milk

Organic sour cream

½ cup fresh cilantro

½ cup fresh parsley

2 fresh, ripe avocadoes

Instructions:

Heat a large saucepan on medium heat with 2 tablespoons virgin coconut oil. Add onion, garlic, and red bell pepper and sauté for 5 minutes. Then add all three beans; mix well. Add crushed tomatoes and all seasonings, stirring occasionally. Add fresh parsley and cilantro. Cook with lid on for 45 minutes on low heat. Serve with fresh sour cream and fresh avocado.

Eucalyptus

The oil of the eucalyptus plant has a unique flavor and scent and is used for a wide range of medical conditions. Eucalyptus oil is distilled oil that comes from the leaf of the plant. It is used to help relieve symptoms of the common cold and is found in many cough lozenges and inhalants. Eucalyptus oil vapor acts as a decongestant when it is inhaled. It is used to treat bronchitis and other respiratory infections.

This oil has a wide range of useful properties:

- Antiseptic
- Anti-inflammatory
- Deodorant
- Fragrance
- Bug repellent

Eucalyptus is a good remedy to have in your medicine cabinet.

Rosemary

Rosemary is a wonderfully earthy, aromatic, woodsy-tasting herb that's great for cooking, air fresheners, and aromatherapy. This amazing Mediterranean herb has been used for more than four thousand years for both medicine and food. Physicians and herbalists alike used rosemary for a wide range of ailments. During the fourteenth century, physicians believed that rosemary would protect many from the bubonic plague that killed thirty-eight thousand Londoners, making rosemary an expensive herb.

Consider rosemary one of your nutritionally power-packed spices. Not only does rosemary have a pretty name, but she's full of life-giving properties.

Sage

Sage is the sister herb of the rosemary plant and has also been used for thousands of years for medicinal and spiritual purposes. Sage is a desert herb with an aromatic sent. It is native to the Mediterranean. Some people compare the aroma of burning sage to marijuana. Burning sage or *smudging* is a purification ritual used to cleanse people or an area from negative energies. Sage can be found fresh, ground, or as an essential oil.

Fresh or dried sage is a lovely herb to enhance roasted vegetables or use as a scent to refresh the house.

Dill

Dill is popular in my home since my husband is from Ukraine and dill weed is used in many Ukrainian dishes. Dill weed is used fresh as well, as a condiment spice, and has a sweet yet anise flavor, great for sautéed dishes and stews. Dill is wonderful on fresh salads and hot soups to add a unique bite.

The word dill comes from the Norwegian word *dilla*, meaning to soothe, yet dill weed is native to Russia. Dill weed has been used as both food and medicine for more than four thousand years and is used today for its antimicrobial properties and its protective health benefits against free radicals and carcinogens. Today, dill is known in the holistic industry as a *chemo-protective* food since it neutralizes many types of cancer-causing elements found in charcoal smoke and other environmental toxins known to cause cancer.

> *For dill is not threshed with a threshing sledge, nor is the cartwheel driven over cumin; But dill is beaten out with a rod and cumin with a club.*
>
> — Isaiah 28:27 NAS

Thyme

Thyme has been a superstar herb for thousands of years dating back to the Roman era. Thyme was an antidote for poison and a symbol for bravery in battle. It has a distinctive, minty, earthy taste similar to the taste of licorice and goes well with lamb and chicken dishes. Many culinary chefs have also prepared soups, chowders, and custards using the herb thyme. The oil and leaf are used to soothe coughs and sore throat, alleviate flatulence, and as a diuretic.

Anise Seed

Anise seed is a Mediterranean plant related to the parsley family. All parts of the anise plant were used during ancient and biblical times as medicine and a spice. Anise was first introduced to Europe in the seventeenth century as a spice and fragrance. Anise is not only used for sweet desserts, fragrance, and savory dishes, but also has healing properties that combat digestive issues and low libido, soothes a cough, and helps increase healthy levels of neurochemicals in the brain. Anise seed tastes similar to licorice and fennel.

Cumin

Cumin is a yellow-brown colored herb used widely in Indian and Mexican cuisine. Cumin seeds are used both whole and ground. It has a peppery taste with a slightly citrus overtone and packs a punch of flavor in chili, soups, stews, and sauces.

The ancient Israelites used dried cumin seeds to flavor their food and as medicine. Today, cumin is recognized and used for its medicinal benefits.

Cumin:

- Helps with digestion
- Stimulates lactation
- Improves immunity
- Prevents cardiovascular disease
- Treats urinary disorders
- Reduces fever
- Is high in iron

Cumin is also known for its antimicrobial properties, as well high in anti-inflammatory agents.

> *Does he not level its surface and sow dill and scatter cumin and plant wheat in rows, barley in its place, and rye within its area?*
>
> —Isaiah 28:25 NAS

Aloe

Aloe originated in Northern Africa and its superior medicinal properties have been known for centuries. This tropical plant grows in the United States in Texas, Arizona, and Florida. Aloe is another one of my favorite plants; in fact, I have one growing in the window of my office. Fresh aloe gel directly from the plant is the best way to receive its medicine. Most aloe juices and gels are highly processed to extend their shelf life and thus lose most of their medicinal benefits. Pure aloe directly from the plant is widely used for its healing properties in treating burns and sunburns, preventing scars, healing bruises and skin rashes, and as a wonderful skin moisturizer. Aloe soothes digestion, fight athlete's foot, and softens stretch marks.

Please try my fresh aloe juice recipe for its amazing healing benefits and great taste.

Toni's Tropical Aloe Beverage

Place 2 tablespoons of fresh aloe gel in a blender. Cut 2 oranges into pieces after removing skin and seeds. Add ½ cup fresh pineapple chunks, 1 cup raw coconut water, and ½ teaspoon Ceylon cinnamon. Blend until creamy and enjoy.

Mint

I like to call mint *the candy cane herb*. It is native to Europe, Asia, and Australia and also known as *menthe*. Mint is a genus of plants, including peppermint and spearmint. Fresh mint has been used for centuries to treat digestive issues, whiten teeth, freshen breath, and as a pest repellent. Today mint is widely used medicinally and as a food additive in salads, hot and chilled soups, drinks, and as a garnish. Mint has a cool, fresh flavor and always adds just the right amount of freshness when needed.

Mustard

The mustard seed is the smallest of seeds with the biggest benefits.

Mustard is a cruciferous plant with a pungent, sour, and peppery taste. Its seeds or powdered mustard can be used in a variety of dishes. Mustard seeds are high in selenium, a necessary mineral that treats allergies, asthma, insomnia, and high blood pressure.

I find it amazing that the mustard seed was the subject of one of Jesus' most famous parables. This may be because mustard grew so abundantly in Palestine. Mustard seeds are mentioned in the New Testament and the kingdom of heaven is compared to a grain of mustard seed.

> *He told them another parable: The kingdom of heaven is like a mustard seed, which a man took and planted in his field. Though it is the smallest of seeds, yet when it grows, it is the largest of plants and becomes a tree, so that the birds come and perch in its branches.*
> —Matthew 13:31-32 NIV

> *And Jesus said unto them, Because of your unbelief: for verily I say unto you. If ye have faith as a grain of mustard seed, ye shall say unto this mountain, remove hence to yonder place; and it shall remove; and nothing shall be impossible unto you.*
> —Matthew 17:20 KJV

Frankincense and Myrrh

Frankincense is known as the king of the oils and is described as piney and woodsy with a lemony, yet sweet aroma. Myrrh comes from an Arabic word *murr*, meaning *bitter*, and has a slightly earthy scent that resembles black licorice. In biblical times, myrrh was given to baby Jesus along with frankincense and gold. Frankincense was sold as a spice or an anointing oil and used in the tabernacle. Frankincense was used as a salve for the purification of the dead and burned as a holy incense in Jerusalem's sacred temple.

Both frankincense and myrrh were used in ancient times for their antiseptic and anti-inflammatory properties. Today, they are used successfully in the holistic industry to treat bacterial and fungal infections, parasites, skin problems, and many forms of cancer.

> *They entered the house and saw the child with his mother, Mary, and they bowed down and worshiped him. Then they opened their treasure chests and gave him gifts of gold, frankincense, and myrrh.*
> —Mathew 2:11 NLT

Essential oils are one of God's amazing healing medicines given to us. I believe the personal use of these oils will give you the gift of being healed directly by our loving God.

> *Is anyone among you sick? Let him call for the elders of the church, and let them pray over him, anointing him with oil in the name of the Lord.*
> —James 5:14 ESV

Sources for these herbs can be found in the resource section of this book.

CHAPTER TWENTY

The Truth About Supplements

Have you ever consumed a vitamin supplement that promised you many great things, yet you felt sick to your stomach after you swallowed that pill?

Have you ever thought that mega dosages of supplements will make up for eating junk?

Whether you answer yes or no, this chapter is for you.

Diets of whole, unprocessed foods are critical. Supplements cannot replace the natural foods created by God for our health. Remember the right supplements are important, but they should never take the place of good nutrition. Supplements are supposed to *supplement,* not replace, real food. However, choosing the correct and chemical-free supplements is also important.

I learned this message in a difficult manor.

As you now know, I was once sick. The wrong source of supplements—synthetic vitamins—contributed to my poor health, along with my improper diet. I am sure you have walked around many health food stores reading the back of several bottles, wondering which supplement you should take. I know I did.

All vitamins are not created equal. So many supplements on the market today are synthetic, including some health food store brands.

Vitamins are vital to our health and to the proper functioning of our bodies. A healthy, whole food, organic diet provides nutrients that the body needs, but supplements can ensure that your body receives a healthy serving of specific vitamins. The bottom line is we need these vitamins, whether we get them from our daily diet, from sunshine, or from store-bought capsules, liquids, or powders.

Vitamin deficiencies lead to a wide range of health problems:

- Anorexia
- Obesity
- Organ malfunction
- Different types of cancers
- Confusion
- Depression
- Fatigue

The right supplementation can correct these deficiencies. The deficiency of *one* vitamin can cause a laundry list of health issues while the sufficiency of one vitamin can reverse these conditions.

Synthetic vitamins are human-made products, created in labs. Many vitamins and minerals are manufactured synthetically with chemicals that do not come straight from natural sources. They are designed to *mimic* the way natural vitamins act in our bodies, often resulting in health issues when consumed.

When you consume synthetic supplements, your body cannot recognize the artificial elements. These artificial ingredients can cause health issues, including toxicity.

Natural vitamins are derived directly from plant material containing the actual vitamin, free of chemicals and high processing. They are not produced in a test tube.

Real, minimally processed, whole food supplements can even be taken on an empty stomach since they are actual food-sourced and the body recognizes them as food. Whole food supplements are easily assimilated, metabolized, and used by the body due to their live active enzymes. Enzymes and probiotics, as well as vitamins and minerals, should always be present in the food we eat as well as our supplementation.

Supplements should be from whole food sources to augment a healthy diet.

Nature is whole. When consuming vitamins in natural foods, they are not isolated from other ingredients. Synthetic vitamins are isolated or simulated nutrients that do not account for the phytonutrients present in a whole plant. We are beginning to understand how lesser-known compounds in plants react with each other as we eat them. We have evolved to recognize the whole, not just individual chemicals, that have been created in a lab to approximate an essential vitamin (Brown, 2014).

Synthetic versions of vitamins do not occur in nature and contain chemical compounds that are not for human consumption. We should eat the food we gather from the Earth, not the food we create in a lab. Humanity has been eating whole foods since the inception of time.

Synthetic vitamins are created by a process *unlike* the metabolic processes that plants and animals use to create natural ones. A finished synthetic vitamin is usually a compound designed by humans. These synthetic vitamins are not as bioavailable, absorbable, or usable by the body. They are not what we find in natural food. They are difficult on the kidneys and are often considered toxins.

Imposter Vitamins

A good first rule is to avoid supplements that use words ending in -*acid*, -*ide*, and sometimes –*ate*, or that use the *dl* before the name. These are clues that your supplement contains synthetic vitamins. Be aware that some medical doctors may prescribe these forms of supplementation for you.

Here is a list of vitamins that should be avoided at all cost in their synthetic form:

- Vitamin A: retinyl palmitate or retinyl acetate
- Vitamin B1 (thiamine): thiamine mononitrate, thiamine hydrochloride
- Vitamin B2 (riboflavin): synthetic riboflavin
- Vitamin B3 (niacin): nicotinic acid
- Vitamin B5 (pantothenate): pantothenic acid
- Vitamin B6 (pyridoxine): pyridoxine hydrochloride
- Vitamin B9 (folate): folic acid
- Vitamin B12 (cobalamin): cyanocobalamin
- Choline: choline chloride, choline bitartrate
- Vitamin C: ascorbic acid
- Vitamin D: irradiated ergosteral, calciferol
- Vitamin E: dl-alpha tocopherol, dl-alpha tocopherol acetate or succinate
- Biotin: d-Biotin
- PABA (not a true vitamin): para-aminobenzoic acid

Instead, search for natural sources of these vitamins in foods and in supplements.

Natural Vitamin A

Vitamin A is present in food as beta-carotene. The body converts this compound into vitamin A. Vitamin A can be toxic in large doses. Beta-carotene is a natural safeguard against the toxicity that leads to organ damage.

Sources natural sources of vitamin A:

- Green, leafy vegetables
- Beef liver
- Carrots
- Sweet potatoes
- Butter

Natural Vitamin B1

Thiamin, or vitamin B1, is a water-soluble vitamin created by plants and bound to phosphate. Digestion releases the thiamin using specialized enzymes that target phosphate. Synthetic vitamins are often crystalline and cause damage and mineral accumulation where it isn't needed (Brown, 2014).

Some natural sources of vitamin B1:

- Beef
- Nuts
- Oats
- Legumes
- Eggs
- Yeast

Natural Vitamin B2

Riboflavin is easily absorbed, is involved in energy metabolism, and promotes iron absorption. Unnatural sources of B2 are not easily absorbed and are expelled with urine like a toxin.

Some natural sources of B2:

- Spinach
- Beet greens
- Lamb
- Milk
- Beef liver
- Broccoli

Natural Vitamin B3

Vitamin B3 is commonly called *niacin*. Niacin can have side effects which may include a rushed heat sensation, but these are minimal when coming from plant foods (Brown, 2014).

Some natural sources of B3 are:

- Yeast extract
- Bran
- Lamb liver
- Fish
- Green Peas
- Avocado

Natural Vitamin B5

Pantothenate is the natural version of this essential B vitamin. Our bodies need B5 to synthesize and metabolize proteins, carbohydrates, and fats.

Some natural sources of Vitamin B5 are:

- Mushrooms
- Liver
- Egg yolks
- Sunflower seeds
- Salmon

Natural Vitamin B6

B6, *pyridoxine*, is used by the body for metabolism, maintaining hormone levels, and hemoglobin formation. Synthetic forms of this vitamin come from petroleum products and can actually inhibit the action of natural B6 in the body.

Some natural sources of B6 are:

- Fish
- Organ meats
- Starchy vegetables
- Non-citrus fruits

Natural Vitamin B7

Biotin is involved in cell growth, fat production, and metabolism.

Some natural sources of B7 are:

- Organ meats
- Barley
- Yeast
- Corn
- Eggs
- Milk
- Avocado

Natural Vitamin B9

This B vitamin exists in food as *folate*. It plays a vital role in the creation and repair of DNA, thus this vitamin is vital before and during pregnancy. Folic acid doesn't exit naturally in foods and doesn't absorb easily into the body.

Some natural sources of B9 are:

- Citrus fruits
- Bananas
- Cantaloupes
- Barley

Natural Vitamin B12

Cobalamin, B12, is a water-soluble vitamin that is essential for DNA synthesis, brain and nervous system function, and red blood cell formation. Vitamin B12 is also necessary for the breakdown of homocysteine and cardio-reactive proteins, which are both associated with cardiovascular disease. The human body does not create B12 and must obtain it through dietary sources. It is only produced by certain bacteria. It is most readily available to humans through animal products. Vegans needs to seek a safe, natural supplement to ensure they receive enough of this vital vitamin.

Some natural sources for B12 are:

- Liver
- Salmon
- Mackerel
- Beef
- Eggs
- Fish

- Liver
- Raw-milk cheese
- Poultry

Plant-based sources include:

- Nuts
- Seeds
- Fruit
- Vegetables
- Grains
- Legumes

Natural Vitamin C

This vitamin is readily available in citrus, red bell peppers, berries, and many fruits and vegetables. In nature it is combined with flavonoids and phytonutrients that help in its absorption and use. This vitamin is extremely easy to obtain in our diet (Brown, 2014). Ascorbic acid often comes from genetically modified corn, so stick to natural sources.

Natural Vitamin D

The human body actually creates vitamin D itself, so it's technically not a vitamin. About twenty minutes of sunlight a day allows our bodies to produce all that we need.

Natural Vitamin E

Vitamin E is a fat-soluble vitamin, that is actually a group of compounds that protect fats from oxidation. The most biologically active form is found in grains, seeds, and the oils from grains and seeds (Brown, 2014).

Natural Vitamin K

This vitamin plays a key role in proper blood clotting. It is primarily found in dark green, leafy vegetables, such as kale, spinach, Swiss chard, parsley, and turnip greens. Synthetic forms of this vitamin are derived from hydrogenated soybean oil, a bad idea in many ways.

A Note on Calcium

Be aware of calcium supplements that may come from rocks and shells. *Calcium carbonate* and *calcium citrate* are popular forms of calcium. These calcium derivatives are removed from rocks and shells and may calcify in several areas of your body.

Calcium can build up in places where it normally doesn't occur in the body. Over time, these deposits may harden, disrupting normal processes.

Since calcium is transported through the bloodstream, calcification can occur in almost any part of the body:

- Calcifying in the arteries contributes to hardening of the arteries.

- Calcifying of the eyes contributes to cataracts.

- Calcifying in the joints and tendons contributes to arthritis and brittle bones, which may lead to osteoporosis.

- Calcifying of the brain, characterized as either abnormal deposits of calcium or cranial calcification, may contribute to a stroke.

- Calcifying in the organs potentially causes kidney stones and gallstones.

There may be many forms of calcium provided by the Earth but the only form of calcium fit for human and animal consumption is from plants. Perhaps this is the reason why milk was once considered a calcium-rich food. When cows graze on green pasture, the milk they provide is *liquid grass.*

Your calcium supplement should be whole food, plant-form.

The advantages to choosing plant-form calcium over rock and shell source calcium are endless. Plants from nature are the preferred source of nutrients for the body. I've said that many times, right?

Consider that plant-based calcium supplements contain dozens of naturally occurring minerals and trace elements, such as magnesium, silica, boron, vanadium, and strontium—all linked to healthy bones. In addition, there are a wide variety of whole food vitamins and minerals, live probiotics, enzymes, and vitamin D that increase the absorption of calcium.

Minerals come from the Earth so they are not classified as *organic,* but plants incorporate minerals and combine them with organic compounds. Therefore, minerals should also be obtained from whole foods. This is how our bodies recognize, incorporate, and utilize them into our systems. Minerals often combine with proteins to form enzymes.

Your body is begging you for the vitamins and minerals it knows, loves, and needs. The best sources can only be found in whole food supplements.

Enzymes

Enzymes are substances produced by living organisms that act as a catalyst for specific biochemical reactions. These reactions help us break down and digest fats, carbohydrates, and proteins so they can be metabolized optimally during the digestive process and then eliminated properly.

Probiotics

Probiotics are live organisms that come from real, live, fermented food, bringing life to our bodies and supporting immune function. Probiotics have the unique ability to destroy unfriendly microbes in the digestive tract that result in disease.

Think of is this way: pro means *for* and bio means *life*.

It is vital to consume cultured foods for their high probiotic content. Probiotics infiltrate the gut with friendly bacteria, leaving unfriendly bacteria no room to survive. Probiotics are critical for gut health, which, in turn, is responsible for a healthy immune system. Probiotics come in many strains and species.

Which ones are best for you?

First, the best way to add probiotics is to consume raw, lacto-fermented foods. These foods include:

- Raw, lacto-fermented sauerkraut
- Kombucha
- Whole, raw kefir
- Whole yogurt

For information on supplementation of probiotics, please refer to the list below.

L. acidophilus—this species colonizes the wall of the small intestine, as well as aids the digestion of dairy foods. This is the most important strain of the *lactobacillus* family.

B. longum — similar to L. *acidophilus* — this probiotic strain is beneficial to the survival of the gut wall lining. *B. longum* is highly effective in retarding growth of unfriendly and harmful bacteria. This species is commonly found in the digestive tracts of adults.

B. bifidum — this is found in the small and large intestines, another necessary strain for the digestion of dairy products. *B. bifidum* is also known for the breakdown and assimilation of carbohydrates, fats, and proteins.

L. fermentum — this *lactobacillus* strain helps promote a healthy level of gut bacteria in the intestines, creating a balanced environment.

L. rhamnosus — this strain is brilliant at recognizing unfriendly, foreign species of bacteria, which can cause traveler's diarrhea.

Supplementation of these strains can be found in powders, liquids, and capsules.

Look for clues on your vitamin's label that offer insight into the origin of the vitamin.

With any meal plan or healthy eating regimen, you must always go back to nature for optimal nutrition benefit. This truth also pertains to supplementation. Once again, to obtain great health and heal your body, learn to recognize the ingredients you are consuming.

My suggestions of whole food supplements can be found in the resource section of this book.

CHAPTER TWENTY-ONE

What's Cooking America?

All About Cookware

If you love cooking like I do, then you may wonder which cookware is safe for you and your loved ones. If you're not wondering, then you should be. There are many dangerous products out there being promoted as healthy. I have witnessed people cooking healthy, wonderful meals in the unhealthiest cookware. That's defeating the purpose, so let's examine why.

Nonstick cookware is in the kitchens of 90 percent of American households. This popular cookware is one of the most dangerous. Its toxic elements leach into your food as soon as heat is applied. There is absolutely nothing healthy about nonstick cookware. For instance, Teflon and *perfluorooctanoic acid* (PFOA) are two known carcinogens lurking in your nonstick cookware. These two caustic poisons increase your risk for digestive disorders, flu-like systems, brain and neurological issues, and thyroid, ovarian, and prostate cancers.

If you have been cooking in nonstick cookware, then your family may have PFOA in their blood. It has been estimated that 95 percent of Americans, including children, have PFOA in their blood. Every time you use nonstick cookware, the heat allows this toxic disease-forming poison to leach into your food.

"In retrospect, this may seem like one of the biggest, if not the biggest, mistakes the chemical industry has ever made," said Jane Houlihan, vice president for research at the Environmental Working Group, an activist organization. "And how could they not be in our blood?" (Jockers, 2011)

The Environmental Protection Agency (EPA) has also revealed that PFOA poses developmental and reproductive risks to our bodies.

Animal studies (Jockers, 2011) have linked the chemical to:

- Risks of liver, pancreatic, testicular, and mammary gland tumors
- Altered thyroid hormone
- Damage to the immune system
- Reproductive difficulties
- Infertility and birth defects

Crockpots, Slow Cookers, and Pressure Cookers

The main health concerns with crockpots and slow cookers are lead, aluminum, and cadmium.

Cadmium is a toxic metal commonly found in cookware and industrial paints. Cadmium is a potential cause for a variety of serious health concerns. Inhalation exposure can result in flu-like symptoms, chills, fever, muscle pain, and possible damage to the lungs. The EPA considers cadmium a carcinogen.

Aluminum is a nonmagnetic, ductile metal. Aluminum is used in deodorants and hair and skin products. Exposure can lead to problems, such as Alzheimer's disease, digestive issues, and many forms of cancer.

Lead is a heavy post-transition chemical element. There is no such thing as *safe* lead. The health risks of lead are high for all of us, and lead is especially harmful to children, who absorb a higher proportion per body weight and are more vulnerable to its effects.

The Mayo Clinic has stated that "lead poisoning occurs when lead builds up in the body, often over a period of months or years. Even small amounts of lead can cause serious health problems" (Mayo Clinic, 2016).

One serving of food prepared using contaminated cookware won't kill you, but over the years it will have an accumulated effect on your bodily systems. This effect could lead to lead poisoning, which is linked to a wide number of neurological problems. In children, lead poisoning is linked to learning disabilities, damage to connective brain tissue, developmental delays, and lower IQ scores.

Slow Cooker Brands and Lead Contamination

The following list was compiled by Kelley Herring, Healing Gourmet:

1. Vita Clay: This unglazed earthenware was independently tested and found to be 99.9 percent lead free.

2. Elite Gourmet Quart Transparent Slow Cooker: Insert is glass, so there's no known risk of lead exposure.

3. Precise Heath 12-inch Surgical Stainless Steel Deep Electric Skillet/Slow Cooker: Insert is surgical grade stainless steel, so no known risk of lead.

4. Proctor Silex: States there is no lead or cadmium in the crock.

5. Kitchen Aid: states their slow cooker glazes are lead-free.

6. Sunpentown S-5355 Zisha Slow Cooker: Sunpentown contains a clay insert and states that is it lead free.

7. Crockpot and Rival: States their product meets FDA guidelines for lead.

8. Cuisinart: States their slow cooker glazes are lead-free.

9. Hamilton Beach: States that they satisfy FDA heavy metal requirements.

10. West Bend: States that glazes are inspected for maximum allowable amounts of trace elements in accordance with United States Food and Drug Administration's guidelines. Keep in mind, if the glazes are chipped or cracked, the vessel should not be used (Herring, 2014).

The Safest Materials in Cookware

Cast iron: an iron alloy carbon readily cast in a mold. Pure cast iron has been safely used for centuries. Eating food cooked in cast iron contributes to a healthy immune system. You can receive your iron intake from cooking in cast iron cookware. This vital mineral is crucial for maintaining healthy energy levels.

Stainless steel: an iron alloy containing chromium, resistant to tarnishing and rust. Stainless steel is durable and resistant to scratches and easy to clean. It is easy to maintain and has a beautiful appearance. This material is a safe alternative to nonstick cookware.

Clay pots: a traditional way of cooking. The benefits of this natural cookware include a reduction of acidity in foods since clay pots are slightly alkaline. Clay pots gradually circulate steam and moisture, creating an evenly cooked meal. Clay is a natural substance of earth and soil found in areas where streams or rivers flowed. The breakup and remains of flora and minerals pulverize into particles called clay.

Ceramic: an inorganic nonmetallic solid of either metal or nonmetal compounds that have been hardened and shaped using high heat temperatures. The word ceramic comes from the Greek word *pottery*. Be aware that some so-called ceramic cookware may contain synthetic coatings, such as aluminum, arsenic, and other toxic metals that can leach into your food.

Safe Coffee Makers

In my opinion, there's nothing like the old-fashioned percolator. Coffee is supposed to be perked and brewed to perfection, not automatically dripped. Most automatic drip makers are made with aluminum, plastic, and lead, leaching directly into your cup.

Nontoxic coffee makers:

1. Presto 02811 12-cup stainless coffee and tea makers
2. Chemex 8-cup all glass, lead-free coffee maker
3. Primula stainless steel stovetop espresso maker
4. Hamilton Beach D50065 commercial 60-cup stainless steel coffee urn
5. Breville BDC550XL The You Brew Glass Drip Coffee Maker
6. West Bend classic stainless steel percolator

Nontoxic coffee filters:

1. Osaka stainless steel reusable filter
2. Chemex bonded unbleached pre-folded square coffee filters
3. If You Care unbleached brown coffee filters

Nontoxic pressure and slow cookers:

1. Presto pressure cooker
2. Vita Clay Smart Organic multi-cooker
3. Instant Pot Lux60
4. Delonghi DCP707 stainless steel programmable 5-quart slow cooker
5. Prestige stainless steel pressure cooker

Frying pans, pots, and baking pans:

1. Dr. Mercola Healthy Chef cookware and Healthy Ceramic cookware
2. Lodge cast–iron cookware
3. Fox Run stainless muffin pan
4. Green pan
5. Cuisinart MCP 12N MultiClAD pro stainless steel 12-piece cookware set
6. Heim Concept 12-piece stainless steel cookware set
7. Chalphalon Classic stainless steel cookware set, 10-pieces
8. Miriam's Eastern Cookware/ Miriam's Earthen cookware clay pots
9. Emile Henry cookware

Juicers, blenders, and food processors:

1. Vitamix blenders
2. Kitchenaid food processor
3. Breville juicer

4. Hurom juicer
5. Nutribullet and Nutribullet RX
6. Immersion hand blender
7. Jack LaLanne power juicer *pro*
8. Norwalk juicer
9. Kitchenaid Diamond blender
10. Juicepresso cold-press juicer

Microwave Dangers

The microwave has become a popular kitchen appliance within the last forty years. Unfortunately, many overlook its potential dangers, as it provides a fast meal. This convenient devise destroys the DNA in food and therefore the body cannot recognize it, making it difficult to digest.

Whatever you put into the microwave suffers the same destructive process. If you only use the microwave to heat up water, the microwave still disrupts the molecules in the water. They move more rapidly, effecting our health. This movement causes friction, which denatures the original design of the substance. These disrupted molecules are nonexistent in nature.

Since the body cannot recognize these foreign substances, it surrounds itself in fat cells to protect itself from the dead food. Keep in mind that microwaving your food causes up to 97 percent of the nutrient content to be lost. The electromagnetic frequencies that are emitted through microwaving become airborne, contributing to DNA damage that leads to cancer.

How the Microwave Works

The microwave is a form of non-ionizing radiation that alters the electromagnetic nature of atoms. The process is similar to

CT scans and mammograms. Typically, your microwaved food is being zapped by high frequency waves of heat. This process is considered a rapid force of extreme heat in a short period of time, which denatures the molecular structure of the food.

The results are damaged and oxidized nutrients that cannot properly be digested. Antioxidants are destroyed, yet these are the most critical of the nutrients for the prevention of disease. The body is electrochemical in nature and any force that disrupts that system will greatly affect the physiology of the body, resulting in disease over time.

One Final Thought

We are all busy these days, and I understand that issue more than you know. However, jeopardizing our health isn't worth a quickly zapped meal. I believe that we all fall into the rut of rushing and cutting corners, but our health should come first.

My advice is to remove the microwave from your home so there is no temptation to use the toxic device. Throwing it out the window may be a thought, but it's not a safe or wise option. Use a toaster oven, which will heat your food at a normal pace and without the electromagnetic and radioactive pollution. Your best choice would be to consume more raw foods and manage your time more efficiently. Using the oven and stove top the way we all did before microwaves is a possible and wise choice.

Our Furry Friends

We don't want to forget our four-legged, furry friends. If you are an animal lover like me, then you must be wondering what the best food is for your best friend. Giving our animals the best food, a warm bed, lots of toys, and mega dosages of love is the recipe for a happy, healthy pet.

Loving our cats and dogs is easy, but finding the best food source can present a problem. We must first understand that animals, like humans, should consume the foods of their ancestors. Whole, organic, mostly raw and unprocessed are the characteristics of a healthy canine and feline diet. Dogs are descended from the wolf *Canis lupus*, and the cat's ancestors are of the species called *Felis sylvestris*, the African wildcat. If you named your kitty Sylvester, then you were right on. The feeding behavior of both cats and dogs should be based on their roots.

Most commercial pet foods are loaded with chemicals and artificial ingredients that are contributing to most of the health issues in animals today. Allergies are an epidemic in dogs and cats, and these allergies are linked right back to their meals and treats. As with any food source, we should be choosing organic for our four-legged friends. Keeping their bodies free of pesticides and genetically modified ingredients is critical for optimal health—no different than humans.

Purchasing organic pet foods is a step in the right direction. However, these foods are still processed, much like boxed cereals. Kibbles are highly processed foods, extruded at high temperatures. The high heat process damages any nutritional value, making the food difficult for your pet to digest. Keep in mind that all disease begins in the gut, so a healthy gut is a healthy immune system. Bad pet food sources are contributing to inflammatory conditions, including digestive disorders, thyroid issues, diabetes, and many types of cancers.

What to Feed Your Pet

Know well the condition of your flocks and pay attention to your herds.
— Proverbs 27:23 NAS

There are so many different types of dog and cat foods on the market today: high protein, low carbohydrate, holistic, grain-free, and raw.

How much more confusing can it get?

In my opinion, the perfect pet food doesn't exist.

In the wild, cats focus mainly on what to hunt rather than what to eat while they modify their food preference based on experience. Dogs as wolves hunted their food pretty much in the same fashion as the wild cat. Dogs and cats are omnivorous by nature, meaning they eat from both plant and animal kingdoms. As with humans, our pets need to obtain and maintain great health by relying on whole, organic food sources.

Here are the top characteristics when looking for the best pet food:

- Be sure your food source is organic and free of animal and vegetable by-products.

- Be sure your brand is free of a generic name since generic brands usually contain the highest levels of chemicals and synthetic vitamins.

- Be sure your pet food is lower in grains and free of artificial coloring, flavoring, and preservatives that result in allergies and other sicknesses.

- Be sure your pet food contains healthy fats that are critical for healthy digestion, energy, and optimal bone, brain, and heart function.

- Be sure your pet food is packed with essential vitamins and minerals.

Keep these principles as guidelines. You can either make your own or use these guides to find the best quality pet food out there today. I make my own dog food for my beautiful furry friend, Peanut, a golden retriever.

I purchase pasture-fed meats from humanely raised farms and prepare them in healthy, unrefined oils like extra virgin coconut oil and a bit of Celtic salt and organic veggies. Peanut is a happy, healthy boy.

Don't forget dessert. Peanut absolutely loves raw carrots and has them every day instead of commercial dog biscuits and treats. You may also want to drizzle extra virgin olive oil on top of the food right before they chow down. Adding probiotics and vitamins to your pet's foods is also a wonderful way to supplement their diet. Making and storing a container of healthy meats and veggies with the best unrefined oils and salt for the week is a great way to save time.

You will notice your pet becoming happier and healthier, with a shinier coat.

Additional foods for dogs:

- Blueberries
- Carrots
- Pumpkin
- Sweet potatoes
- Watermelon

- Apples
- Eggs
- Oats

Until one has loved an animal, a part of one's soul remains unawakened.

— Anatole France

A righteous man has regard for the life of his animal, but even the compassion of the wicked is cruel.

— Proverbs 12:10 NAS

CHAPTER TWENTY-TWO

Marketing Strategies

Congratulations! You have almost made it through this entire book, and you have learned a lot about the dangers of the modern food industry and how it affects your health. You have also learned the benefits of real, whole, unprocessed, organic foods and their connection to God's word through scripture. It is now time for you to discover the truth about many marketing strategies and how they influence your health.

Don't be a victim of these deceiving marketing strategies that are lurking at your local grocery store. We are overfed, undernourished, and deficient.

The Labels

All-natural. These words are one of the most deceiving marketing strategies of all time. They mean simply that ingredients came from nature at one time. All-natural products can be virtually anything that once came from nature. These impostors are genetically modified, full of pesticides, made with corn syrup and maltodextrin, as well as additives, preservatives, and artificial ingredients. Most *all-natural* products are also highly processed: pasteurized, ultra-pasteurized, homogenized, refined, adulterated, and may even be bleached.

Fat-free. Foods labeled fat-free are usually high in sugar and most likely chemical laden. These chemicals are often hydrolyzed corn starch from genetically modified corn, which usually includes monosodium glutamate (MSG). Most fat-free foods contain fat-mimicking chemicals that can cause headaches, intestinal cramps, gas, bloating, and diarrhea. They can contribute to weight gain since these chemicals trick your body into eating more.

Light. Food labeled as *light* is once upon a time whole food that has had necessary nutrients and valuable substances removed. This process makes these *lighter* foods unrecognizable to the body. These types of foods are usually fat-free/sugar-free and promoted as healthier choices. Instead, light foods are nothing but chemically processed, nutrient-less, allergy forming, *diet* products. When you consume *fat-free* foods, you'll soon begin to crave carbohydrates to make up for nutrient-deficiency. Turning real food into lighter versions will make you heavier in the long term.

100% juice. This juice may not contain added sugar; however, the juice is normally pasteurized to extend its shelf life for profit. Pasteurization boils the juice at a high temperature, turning the juice into sugar, making your natural sugarless drink a highly inflammatory beverage or liquid candy. I call this sugar-coated marketing.

Sugar-free. Most sugar-free products are *diet* products that contain artificial sweeteners created in a lab. These sweeteners are genetically engineered; they trick your body into hunger, which makes you gain weight. Artificial sweeteners dull your taste buds, making you crave sugar. As you know, eating sugar results in hormonal imbalances, digestive issues, diabetes, and has been linked to many types of cancers.

Fortified. This word appears when naturally occurring vitamins have been chemically removed and synthetic supplementation has been added. These synthetics can include zinc oxide, ascorbic acid, calcium pantothenate, and calcium carbonate, which are all produced from formaldehyde and genetically modified organisms. Furthermore, these synthetic supplements are the cheap forms of nutrients, and your body cannot recognize or utilize them.

Refined. These grains are missing the fiber, bran, germ, and key nutrients due to the milling and grinding process. This significantly modifies the grain from its natural unrefined state, making the grain more difficult to digest.

Enriched. Refined grains that are highly processed with chlorine, bleach, and artificial vitamins are known as enriched. Perfect examples of enriched and fortified products are:

- Pasta
- White rice
- Boxed cereal
- *Whole grain* bread
- White bread
- Crackers
- Cookies
- English muffins
- Bagels

During the processing of the grain, virtually all B vitamins are removed, plus most of the minerals, the fiber, and the good fat, leaving you with a starchy, highly refined product with little nutritional value. The flour that is used in these products is highly refined and processed with chemical agents, making these foods culprits for allergies, asthma, serious digestive issues, and learning disabilities.

Technically, most flours are bleached, whether they are labeled bleached flour or unbleached flour. The differing processes of bleaching sets these two types of flour apart. Bleached flour is treated with toxic chemical agents to speed up aging while unbleached flour is bleached naturally as it ages. Bleached flour uses bleaching agents like benzoyl peroxide and chlorine gas to speed up the flour's aging process.

Yes, I know exactly what you're thinking as you read this — another reason why so many people are sick. This process results in whiter, finer-grain flour with a softer, powdery texture so you can make a nice fluffy loaf of bread or muffins for your loved ones. Unbleached flour bleaches naturally over time from the chemical agents that are added to the flour, making unbleached flour another deceiving marketing strategy and unhealthy option. Don't be deceived by the words *unbleached flour*.

Gluten free. What exactly does this mean? If it's not a naturally occurring gluten-free ancient grains likes millet, brown rice, buckwheat, quinoa, and amaranth, then it probably contains genetically modified potato, corn, or soy flours, which are nothing but chemical-laden, disease-forming, inflammatory substances. These products often also contain refined sugar and canola oil, a genetically modified oil that robs the body of magnesium and vitamin E, two critical nutrients necessary for a healthy heart.

Children's Foods

Children are especially vulnerable to foods, which are marketed with colorful icons to capture the minds of little ones. These food-like products are promoted as *healthy* choices consisting of less sugar or low fat. However, these products often contain more artificial ingredients, chemical additives, and artificial coloring. These poor choices lead to learning disabilities, behavioral and developmental problems, allergies, and asthma.

Organic Labeling

Be cautious about a label that says *made with organic ingredients* because this means only 70 percent of the ingredients are organic and the rest may be pesticide-laden and genetically modified. Keep in mind that products with less than 70 percent organic ingredients may list organically produced ingredients on the side panel of the package, but may not make any organic claims on the front of the package.

If a product is labeled organic without the USDA seal, then 95 percent of the ingredients are organic and the other five percent may contain pesticides. If a product is labeled USDA organic, then the product contains 100 percent organic ingredients, and this is the labeling to guarantee you that your food is 100 percent organic.

Organic means free of chemical fertilizers and genetic engineering.

Don't be fooled by the non-GMO label. It does mean that the product is free of genetically modified organisms; however, this label does not mean the product is organic. The product will still contain chemical fertilizers. The only label that assures 100 percent organic and non-GMO is the organic USDA seal.

Please stop buying packaged nut milks, including coconut and rice milk. I am not saying that nut milks are unhealthy. I am saying the packaged versions are simply not good for you since they are pasteurized, destroying all the nutritional benefit.

Pasteurization means the product is heated at high temperatures, extending the shelf life for profit. There are many chemical-laden ingredients in these products, including artificial vitamins that have the potential to cause sickness. Even the organic nut milks are valueless due to processing methods, so please make your own. Making nut milk is a simple and healthier option. Often there aren't any nuts in the store versions of nut milk, yet *carrageenan*, a suspected cancer-causing ingredient, is added to most brands as a thickener.

Carrageenan is derived from red algae or seaweed. This additive is processed through an alkaline process to produce what many consider to be an *all-natural* food ingredient. It doesn't stop there. This seaweed is prepared in an acidic solution, producing what is called *degraded carrageenan* or *poligeenan*. This form of seaweed is known for its inflammatory properties.

Carrageenan is also used in prescription drug trials to create an inflammatory effect and other health conditions in laboratory animals. This toxic ingredient is used in other products as well, such as cold cuts, baby formula, nut milks, dairy products, pharmaceutical medicine, and as a food additive. Carrageenan is a highly inflammatory additive that results in many inflammatory health conditions when consumed and should be avoided at all cost.

Make your own delicious nut milk by following my simple recipe.

Raw Almond Milk Recipe

Soak approximately ½ cup of raw, organic almonds overnight. (Soak nuts in 2 cups water overnight or 8 hours.) Drain, then add 3–4 cups of pure water or raw coconut water and blend in a high-speed mixer until desired consistency. Add sweetener of choice, preferably organic maple syrup. I like to add organic vanilla extract as well. You can add a pinch of unrefined Celtic salt. Blend and strain. Store your final product in a glass bottle inside the refrigerator for up to eleven days.

You may double ingredients for more milk. You can also follow this same exact recipe and use any other type of nuts for a variety of nut milks.

Maltodextrin is a cheap artificial additive used as a sugar that is mostly from genetically engineered corn. It is added to yogurts, nut milks, gum, sweeteners, supplements, and baked goods. Overconsumption of this additive may cause irritability, nervousness, insomnia, digestive upset, and diarrhea. Long-term use of maltodextrin may cause more severe health conditions.

Keep in mind that real, unprocessed foods are the right ingredients, and real food does not require marketing strategies.

CHAPTER TWENTY-THREE

Recipes for Wellness

A Prescription for SICKNESS

Get all your vaccinations. Vaccinations are a controversial issue in modern medicine. Even though the majority of the conventional medical community believes that vaccines are means of *preventive medicine*, there is a rapidly growing community that strongly disagrees. There is a direct correlation between the toxic ingredients in vaccines and recurring sickness. Through vaccination, we are trading sickness for sickness in both humans and animals.

Vaccines offer artificial immunity, which confuses and bombards the immune system, resulting in immunological damage. Vaccines are not intended to work the way the immune system was designed. Vaccinations do not immunize, they compromise.

Next, eat the foods of modern civilization. Consume conventional, hormone-laden, drugged up, pasteurized, homogenized, genetically modified, fat-free, sugar-free, hydrogenated, prepackaged, refined, artificially fortified, and processed food-like products. Use artificial sweeteners, eat lots of refined sugar, swim in chlorinated pools, use toxic hair and skin care products, cook in nonstick cook ware, never smile or laugh, use antibacterial soaps, remove *unnecessary* body parts, and receive modern dental work, such as amalgam fillings, root canals, and fluoride treatments.

Use the microwave, never open a window, don't exercise, go to bed late, harbor anger and un-forgiveness, never pray, be ungrateful, speak negatively, never apologize, drink chlorinated water, use sunscreen, avoid the sun, and rely on prescription drugs for your health.

A Prescription for Health and WELLNESS

Eat food in the form God created: organic, whole, unprocessed, unrefined, mostly raw, humanely raised. Drink pure water, make fresh raw juices daily, consume plenty of fresh fruits and veggies, avoid the microwave, take whole food supplements, sleep in complete darkness, oil pull often, receive massages twice a month or more, smile often, enjoy fresh air, exercise daily, forgive others—including yourself—speak positively, give hugs, receive hugs, rescue an animal, practice yoga, grounding, and earthing, play outside, plant something, go to bed before 11:00 p.m., pray often, be thankful, take fellowship with positive, likeminded people, and take care of the Earth.

If you are willing and obedient, ye shall eat the good of the land, but if you resist and rebel you will be devoured by the sword. For the mouth of the Lord has spoken.
—Isaiah 1:19-20 NIV

MEAL PLANS

Raw, Lacto-Fermented Sauerkraut

Raw, lacto-fermented sauerkraut is high in enzymes and probiotics—exactly what is needed for digestion. Whenever you have cooked food on your plate, it is extremely important to add some fresh raw sauerkraut for healthy enzyme delivery. Adding raw sauerkraut to your meals can help avoid gas and bloating. Adding approximately one to two tablespoons or more per day is suggested. This healthy food can be found in the refrigerated section of most health food stores. Look for brands that say both *raw* and *organic*. Regular sauerkraut is highly pasteurized, which defeats our purpose and should be avoided.

Salad Dressings

Be creative and use extra virgin cold-pressed olive oil, unrefined flaxseed oil, coconut vinegar, or Bragg's apple cider vinegar, organic spices, such as organic garlic powder and organic onion powder, and fresh-squeezed lemon. Use Celtic or any unrefined salt and black pepper. Add nuts and seeds. Have fun being creative; I believe there's a great chef in all of us.

First Suggestion

Start slow: chew your food well, as digestion begins in the mouth not in the gut. Baby steps! Eating too quickly can cause digestive upset when food cannot be broken down and metabolized properly.

Sample Meals

Here are breakfast, lunch, and dinner suggestions following our principles. Use them to make your journey easier. The source of your food makes all the difference.

These are examples of what your meals should look like.

Always break your fast in the morning with 12–16 ounces of warm or room-temperature water with 1–2 tablespoons of raw vinegar, and or fresh-squeezed lemon, then followed with a raw juice. Recipes may be found in the juicing section of this book.

- Breakfast: pastured or organic eggs any style cooked in coconut oil, add unrefined salt. One slice of sprouted-grain toast with ghee, organic butter, or raw butter. A forkful or two of raw sauerkraut, or toasted sprouted-grain English muffin with either organic butter or raw nut butter of choice.

- Lunch: wild fish of choice or pasture-raised, organic chicken with brown rice, and fresh roasted veggies. Another choice is a smoothie you can take with you to work or out for the day if you want to avoid eating something unhealthy.

- Dinner: quinoa, mixed sautéed veggies, and a green salad. Add raw sauerkraut for digestion.

- Breakfast: presoaked oatmeal, add organic butter, raw coconut butter, coconut oil, fresh fruit, cinnamon, or raw nuts. You may add anything that's healthy. Sweet choices are coconut sugar, raw honey, or maple syrup.

- Lunch: pasture-raised chicken, steamed veggies, real butter, green salad, homemade dressing.

- Dinner: grass-fed beef stew, sweet potato with real butter and Celtic salt, a side of raw sauerkraut, with fresh avocado.

- Breakfast: eggs any style with raw cheese, sprouted gluten-free bagel with organic butter, or raw nut butter.

- Lunch: green salad, homemade dressing, topped with an organic, soy-free veggie burger.

- Dinner: roasted pasture-raised chicken with sweet potato and real butter, Celtic salt, fermented raw sauerkraut and a green salad with avocado.

- Lunch: grilled pasture-raised organic chicken with raw, lacto-fermented veggies, real butter.

- Dinner: wild fish of choice with sautéed broccoli with garlic and oil, Celtic salt and black pepper to your taste. Add raw, lacto-fermented sauerkraut.

- Lunch: wild salmon, or grass-fed beef, veggie of choice with real butter or green salad with protein, such as hard-boiled eggs, raw cheese, or leftover meat from dinner, with homemade dressing using unrefined oils, coconut vinegar, and organic seasonings.

- Dinner: chicken and veggies, side of raw, lacto-fermented sauerkraut. Add brown rice, or quinoa with butter.

- Lunch alternative: smoothie of choice or eggs with raw sauerkraut and sprouted toast with organic butter.

- Dinner: wild fish cooked in coconut oil, sweet potatoes with real butter and Celtic salt. Add a fresh green salad.

- Lunch: quinoa and veggies or a smoothie of choice.

- Dinner: wild fish of choice with organic brown rice and salad. Or substitute brown rice with sweet potatoes; always cook in extra virgin coconut oil.

- Snack: any organic raw nut butter with banana or fruit of choice.

- Green salad: Two handfuls fresh organic mixed greens of choice, add fresh organic veggies of choice, add raw cheese, homemade dressing.

Smoothies are a great meal replacement and easy way to get all your vital nutrients that bring healing. Smoothie recipes can be found in the juicing and blending section of this book.

Important Principles

Keep food whole and organic.

Eat what was created for food in the form it was created.

Do not consume foods that have been altered from their origin, as this makes it difficult for our bodies to digest and heal. Our bodies cannot recognize altered and processed foods.

Fish should always be wild with scales and fins, never farmed-raised. Human-made pellets fed to farmed fish changes their omega-3 content to omega-6 which makes farmed fish an unhealthy choice.

Juice should always be made raw from organic produce. Never use stored juices. These juices are pasteurized to extend shelf life for profit and are inflammatory.

Foods should always be organic.

Oils should always be organic, extra virgin, and unrefined. Coconut oil is best for cooking. Olive oil, flax, and hempseed oils are best for drizzling on salads.

Salt should be unrefined, such as Celtic salt, Icelandic flake salt, or Himalayan, and vinegar should be raw and organic.

Beef should be grass-fed and finished; eggs and chicken should be pasture-raised or organic.

Butter should be organic or raw. Yogurt, milk, and kefir should always be full fat, organic, and plain. Dairy sources should be certified raw, grass-fed, and humanely raised.

Eat sprouted, sourdough, or Ezekiel-type breads that contain ancient grains, and always use organic or raw butter or organic raw nut butters.

Soak your oats overnight. For instructions and my favorite recipe, see the chapter on grains.

Recipes for Infection, Pain, and Prevention

These recipes are not to take the place of professional medical attention. Please contact your health care provider for proper medical care, as these recipes are to be used for educational purposes only.

Cold and Flu Remedy #1

Crush 3 cloves of organic garlic in a small container and add ⅛ teaspoon cayenne pepper. Mix in raw organic honey. Add 1 teaspoon of this concoction to 6–8 ounces of boiling water 3–4 times daily to soothe and shorten the duration of colds and flu. Store the remainder of the recipe in a glass jar in the refrigerator for up to ten days.

Cold and Flu Remedy #2

Drink 1 tablespoon of raw apple cider vinegar mixed with 4 ounces of room-temperature water 3-4 times daily, and then remain on this same recipe once daily for maintenance.

Raw apple cider vinegar is a natural antibiotic, has anti-inflammatory properties, antifungal, anti-candida, antibacterial, and antiviral properties. Raw apple cider vinegar reduces pain, restores intestinal flora, balances blood glucose levels and blood pressure, regulates hormones, clears skin, purifies blood, and makes a great cleaning product without the caustic chemicals of commercial cleaners.

Cold and Flu Remedy #3

Take 1 teaspoon of pure, organic black elderberry syrup 3 times daily for the duration of the sickness and continue up to two weeks after symptoms cease.

Black elderberry is a potent antioxidant that boosts the immune system, improves vision, improves lung and heart health, dramatically calms cough, and is excellent for both viral and bacterial respiratory infections.

Every Day

Consume 1–2 tablespoons of raw apple cider vinegar daily with 16 ounces of water. Store your vinegar in a cool, dry place.

Always be sure your vinegar is both raw and organic to deliver the life-giving properties it offers. The pasteurized versions are useless since they no longer contain the beneficial bacteria.

Indigestion Remedy

Mix four ounces of warm water (not hot) with 1 teaspoon raw apple cider vinegar. Sip within a minute or two, repeat if necessary.

Keep in mind, drinking icy cold water can suppress immune function for up to six hours.

Cough Remedy

Consume 1 teaspoon of 100 percent pure organic black elderberry syrup up to 3 times daily for up to two weeks. Squeeze the juice from 1 fresh, organic lemon. Add 1 teaspoon raw, organic honey, then add 1 tablespoon raw apple cider vinegar. Add ⅛ teaspoon organic cinnamon, 1 teaspoon extra virgin, organic coconut oil. Add 5–8 ounces of boiling hot water and sip as a tea. Consume 2–3 times a day during a cold or flu.

Natural Antibiotic Remedy

Add 4 drops of oregano essential oil to 4 ounces of water, sip slowly 1 or 2 times a day during colds, flu, and bacterial infections.

Headache Remedy

Mix 3-4 drops of each essential oil in a small bowl: peppermint, wintergreen, basil, and frankincense. Massage into temples and behind head, avoiding any contact with eyes.

These oils have a calming effect while reducing inflammation that results in neck and head tension.

Healthcare Product Danger

Please beware of these dangerous, highly toxic, carcinogenic ingredients in most commercial deodorants, skin creams, makeup, hair care products, and toothpaste.

Phthalates – A toxic poison that has been linked to a variety of health issues, including birth defects and cancer.

Triclosan – This chemical is considered a pesticide by the FDA and a carcinogen by the Environmental Protection Agency.

Aluminum – This highly carcinogenic metal has been linked to breast cancer and brain and neurological disorders, such as Alzheimer's disease and dementia.

Fluoride - This neurotoxin can be found in drinking water and in most commercial toothpaste. This toxin has been shown to cause brain and neurological disorders, thyroid conditions, fluorosis of the teeth (brown spots on the enamel of the teeth), and bone cancer.

Parabens – This toxic poison has been known to cause hormonal irregularities that lead to cancer of the thyroid and reproductive organs and to organ toxicity.

Propylene glycol –This toxic poison has the potential to cause seizers, cancer, liver toxicity, and heart disease.

Petroleum by-products – Listed as mineral oil, petrolatum, liquid paraffin, toluene, or xylene, these chemicals are found in many shampoos and soaps. *Dioxin*, a carcinogen, is usually found as an added ingredient along with petroleum by-products.

Lead – It's a potent neurotoxicant and has been found in several popular brands of makeup, including most hair coloring.

Mercury – A neurotoxicant that has the potential to damage human health, mercury — often listed as *thimerosol* — is found in hair color and makeup.

Fragrance – Found in everything from shampoo to deodorant, a single product's secret fragrance mixture can contain potentially hundreds of carcinogenic compounds.

Nan particles – Found in skin creams, shampoos, moisturizers, makeup, and most sunscreens, these toxins are highly carcinogenic and have the potential to destroy human health.

Formaldehyde – As well as preserving dead tissue, this toxin is a hardener in nail polish and even some baked goods. This chemical is a known carcinogen.

Tonijean's Natural Deodorant Recipe

In a small container, add $1/_3$ cup organic extra virgin coconut oil, 2 tablespoons nonaluminum baking soda, 15–20 drops of an essential oil (suggestions: peppermint, lavender, or lemon). Mix well, double ingredients for larger batches. Store in a plastic container for up to 6 months in bathroom cabinet. Use daily.

Tonijean's Homemade Anti-Wrinkle Face Cream

Combine 1½ tablespoon extra virgin coconut oil, 1 teaspoon pure vitamin E oil, 4 drops of geranium oil, 6 drops green tea extract, and 1 tablespoon or more of arrowroot powder. Mix to a spreadable but thick consistency. Store this cream in a sealed plastic container in medicine cabinet for up to 6 months. Double ingredients for more face cream.

Please avoid contact with eyes.

Tonijean's Homemade Toothpaste Recipe

Mix 1–2 teaspoons of organic peppermint essential oil, or spearmint, $\frac{2}{3}$ cup nonaluminum baking soda, 1–2 tablespoons organic extra virgin coconut oil, and ½ teaspoon unrefined sea salt. Keep in small container.

You may store this toothpaste in your medicine chest for up to six months.

Conclusion

I want to thank you for choosing my book and taking your time to read it. I hope that you have gained a wealth of valuable information for yourself and your loved ones. There are many wonderful nutrition guides and programs available in the industry today. Many provide beneficial information, including protein powders, supplements, and diet programs.

As a holistic practitioner, I often witness people reverse their health conditions. These patients work diligently through juicing, preparing their meals, drinking pure water, consuming 100 percent organic foods, taking whole food supplements, practicing forgiveness, speaking positively, exercising, and getting proper rest and sleep. I do believe that these are some of the most important principles to healing and superior health.

I also witness many people who struggle with their health simply because they are not consistent with the right plan. These people are constantly looking for another protein powder or the most recent fad and diet. To experience great health, one must follow the right program, consisting of God's whole, organic foods. There is no program or diet that will ever take the place of real, whole, organic food. Real food is the ingredient to a successful healing regimen.

We Must Eliminate the Cause

We must STOP looking for another magic pill, diet, or protein powder. If you're one of those people searching for another diet plan, another protein powder, or the latest fad, you are still eating human-made, chemical-laden poison, and you're looking for a quick fix.

STOP listening to fads and eat real, whole unprocessed, organic food the way God intended, in the same exact form as ancient and biblical times. I consume the diet of our ancestors, which includes the foods described in this book. I experience extraordinary health every day because of my choices.

These foods are in their original form God created—whole, raw, humanely treated, unprocessed, properly germinated, and organic! Stop listening to man, because there's NOTHING like the infinite wisdom of the Creator and the connection within you. The body cannot heal properly and completely when we are half in and half out. When you exclusively eat real organic, whole food, your body totally heals. When you follow God's plan diligently, your body heals everything. The body doesn't heal selectively by choosing which sickness to heal.

We must stop battling disease and start building wellness. It's that simple.

There's Beauty All Around Us

We may have the power to turn ugliness into beauty. In the end, all living things want peace and love!

Life as we know it has situations that are not always pleasant; we sometimes can't understand why certain things happen. The world is full of evil, but if we look closely enough, we can see beauty and greatness all around us.

If you look deeply enough into bad situations, you will find pain and sadness. People who are so-called bad or evil may be dealing with horror in their lives, but are still here on their journey to carry on.

Regardless of how angry or upset we become when we see unfair situations, it is our responsibility to extend love like Christ did.

When we continue to show love where hate is present, we are creating the chance to turn pain into peace, a victim into victory, tragedies into triumph, a mess into a messenger, sadness into joy, brokenness into wholeness, darkness into light, and hatred into love. We give life where there is death.

Lord, make me an instrument of Thy peace;
Where there is hatred, let me sow love;
Where there is injury, pardon;
Where there is doubt, faith;
Where there is despair, hope;
Where there is darkness, light;
And where there is sadness, joy.
O Divine Master,
Grant that I may not so much seek to be consoled, as to console;
To be understood, as to understand;
To be loved, as to love.
For it is in giving that we receive;
It is in pardoning that we are pardoned;
And it is in dying that we are born to eternal life.
Amen.
—The Prayer of St. Francis of Assisi

A FINAL THOUGHT

You Are the Number One Priority

Taking care of my body is a huge priority in my life. My body is the temple of God our Creator, and it's my spiritual responsibility to take care of my physical body.

Eating food that is unprocessed, pure, clean, organic, and whole is the only source that enters my body.

Experiencing extraordinary health each day is the blessing I receive from consuming God's pharmacy of healing foods.

I choose to reflect health so I can inspire others to do the same.

> *Therefore, I urge you, brothers and sisters, in view of God's mercy, to offer your bodies as a living sacrifice, holy and pleasing to God — this is your true and proper worship.*
> — Romans 12:1 NIV

> *If you listen carefully to the LORD your God and do what is right in his eyes, if you pay attention to his commands and keep all his decrees, I will not bring on you any of the diseases I brought on the Egyptians, for I am the LORD, who heals you.*
> — Exodus 15:26 NIV

Resources

Most of the products listed here can be found in health food stores and some supermarkets, as well as online.

General Websites

BeyondOrganic.com
Eatwild.com
GreenDiary.com
NonGMOShoppingGuide.com
OneGreenPlanet.com
VeganEssentials.com

FOODS AND HEALTH CARE

Cereals
Emmy's Organics: Emmysorganics.com
Erewhon: ErewhonOrganic.com
Food for Life: FoodforLife.com
Lydia's Kind Foods: LydiasKindFoods.com
One Degree Organic Foods: OneDegreeOrganics.com

Chocolate
Raw cacao bars candy: therawchocolatecompany.com

Coconut Water/Kombucha
Earth Circle Organics: EarthCircleOrganics.com
GT's Kombucha: GtsKombucha.com
Harmless Harvest: HarmlessHarvest.com

Cold Cuts; Grass-fed, Pastured Meats

Applegate: Applegate.com (look for products without carrageenan)
Beyond Organic: MyBeyondOrganic.com
Eatwild: Eatwild.com
Nuna Naturals: NunaNatural.com
Nutiva: Nutiva.com
Organic Prairie: OrganicPrairie.com
Weston A. Price: WestonAPrice.org

Cooking Oils, Cold Dish Oils

Bragg: Bragg.com
Dr. Bronner's All-One!: DrBronner.com
Garden of Life: GardenofLife.com
Nutiva: Nutiva.com
Olive Oil Lovers: OliveOilLovers.com
Olivers & Co.: OliviersandCo.com
Papa Vince: PapaVince.com
Tropical Traditions: TropicalTraditions.com

Condiments, Salt, Spices, Extracts

Bragg: Bragg.com
Frontier Co-op: FrontierCoop.com
Great American Spice Company: AmericanSpice.com
Longevity Warehouse: LongevityWarehouse.com
Natierra Himalania Pink Salt: Natierra.com
Real Salt: RealSalt.com
Selina Naturally: SelinaNaturally.com
Simply Organic: SimplyOrganic.com
Sun Organic Farm: SunOrganicFarm.com
Woodstock: Woodstock-Foods.com

Dairy
Ancient Organics: AncientOrganics.com
Butterworks Farm: ButterworksFarm.com
A Campaign for Real Milk: RealMilk.com
Cedar Summit Farm: CedarSummit.com
DITALIA: Ditalia.com (Pecorino Romano grating cheese)
Hawthorne Valley Farm: HawthorneValleyFarm.org
Kalona Super Natural: KalonaSuperNatural.com
Kerrygold: Kerrygold.com
Old Chatham Sheepherding Company:
    OldChathamSheepherding.com
Organic Valley: Organicvalley.com
Pure Indian Foods: PureIndianFoods.com (ghee)
Seven Stars Farm: SevenStarsFarm.com
Traders Point Creamery: TradersPointCreamery.com
Wallaby Yogurt: WallabyYogurt.com
Weston A. Price: WestonAPrice.org

Eggs
Eatwild: Eatwild.com
GrassFed Traditions: GrassFedTraditions.com
The Happy Egg Co.: TheHappyEggCo.com
Vital Farms: VitalFarms.com

Flaxseed/Hemp Seed Oils
Barlean's: Barleans.com
Longevity Warehouse: LongevityWarehouse.com
Nutiva: Nutiva.com
Newman's Own: NewmansOwn.com
Omega Nutrition: OmegaNutrition.com

Flours
Arrowhead Mills: ArrowheadMills.com
Blue Mountain Organics: BlueMountainOrganics.com
Coconut Secret: CoconutSecret.com
Honeyville: Honeyville.com
Now: NowFoods.com
Sunfood Superfoods: Sunfood.com

Grains, Beans, Oats, and Breads
Alvarado Street Bakery: AlvaradoStreetBakery.com
Berlin Natural Bakery: BerlinNaturalBakery.com
Blue Mountain Organics: BlueMountainOrganics.com
Bob's Red Mill: BobsRedMill.com
Eden Foods: EdenFoods.com
Food for Life: FoodforLife.com
Go Raw: GoRaw.com
Jovial: JovialFoods.com
Jyoti Natural Foods: jyotifoods.com
Manna Organics: MannaOrganicBakery.com
Nuts.com: Nuts.com
Now: NowFoods.com
Pure Living: PureLivingOrganic.com
Pure Traditions Foods: Puretraditionsfoods.com
Simple Mills: Simplemills.com
Sun Organic Farm: SunOrganicFarm.com
Tropical Traditions: TropicalTraditions.com
truRoots: truRoots.com

Hummus
Cava: Cavagrill.com
Hope Foods: HopeFoods.com
PTA Pal: PTApal.com

Ice Cream
Aldens Organic: AldensIceCream.com
Raw Ice Cream Company: RawIceCreamCompany.com

NonDairy
Miyoko's Kitchen: miyokoskitchen.com

Non-GMO
Non-GMO Shopping Guide: Nongmoshoppingguide.com

Nut Butters, Coconut Butter
Blue Mountain Organics: BlueMountainOrganics.com
Manna Organics: MannaOrganicBakery.com
Nuts.com: Nuts.com
The Raw Food World: TheRawFoodWorld.com
Artisana Organics: Artisanaorganics.com
Rejuvenative Foods: RejuvenativeFoods.com
Woodstock: Woodstock-Foods.com

Pasta
Explore Cuisine: ExploreCuisine.com
Food for Life: FoodforLife.com
Jovial: JovialFoods.com
King Soba: KingSoba.com
Nature's Legacy: NaturesLegacyforLife.com
Tolerant: TolerantFoods.com
truRoots: truRoots.com

Protein Powders, Bone Broths
Garden of Life: GardenofLife.com
Get Brothed: GetBrothed.com
Longevity Warehouse: LongevityWarehouse.com

Markus Rothkranz Products: MarkusRothkranz.com
Wise Choice Market: WiseChoiceMarket.com

Raw Juice Powders
Garden of Life: GardenofLife.com
Longevity Warehouse: LongevityWarehouse.com
Markus Rothkranz Products: MarkusRothkranz.com
Organifi: Organifi.com
The Raw Food World: TheRawFoodWorld.com

Rice/Quinoa
Eden Foods: EdenFoods.com
Lundberg Family Farms: Lundberg.com (USDA organic and
    sprouted only)
truRoots: truRoots.com

Sauerkraut, Pickles
Eden Foods: EdenFoods.com
Hawthorne Valley Farm: HawthorneValleyFarm.org
Süperkrauts: rawsuperkrauts.com
Woodstock: Woodstock-Foods.com

Snacks
Gnosis Chocolate: GnosisChocolate.com
Go Raw: GoRaw.com
Hail Merry: HailMerry.com
Jackson's Honest: JacksonsHonest.com
Lesser Evil Buddha Bowl Popcorn: LesserEvil.com
Live-Live & Organic: Live-Live.com
Made in Nature dried fruit: MadeinNature.com
Mary's Gone Crackers: MarysGoneCrackers.com
Organic Nectars: OrganicNectars.com

Unique Sprouted Grain Pretzels: UniqueSplits.com
Way Better snacks: GoWayBetter.com
Wonderfully Raw Gourmet Delights macaroons and brownies:
  MyCocoroons.com

Sprouted Nuts and Trail Mixes
Blue Mountain Organics: BlueMountainOrganics.com
Living Intentions: LivingIntentions.com
Organic Living Superfoods: OrganicLivingSuperfoods.com
The Raw Food World: TheRawFoodWorld.com
Sunfood Superfoods: Sunfood.com

Superfoods, Super Herbs
Blue Mountain Organics: BlueMountainOrganics.com
Dragon Herbs: DragonHerbs.com
Hawaiian Organic Noni: Real-Noni.com
Herb Pharm: Herb-Pharm.com
Host Defense Mushrooms: HostDefense.com
Jing Herbs: JingHerbs.com
Living Earth Herbs: LivingEarthHerbs.com
Longevity Warehouse: LongevityWarehouse.com
Markus Rothkranz Products: MarkusRothkranz.com
Mountain Rose Herbs: MountainRoseHerbs.com
Natierra Himalania products: Natierra.com
Nativas Naturals: NativasNaturals.com
Nature's Answer: NaturesAnswer.com
Pure Planet: PurePlanet.com
The Raw Food World: TheRawFoodWorld.com
Sacred Chocolate: SacredChocolate.com
Sunfood Superfoods: Sunfood.com
Wheatgrass Kits: WheatgrassKits.com
Y.S. Eco Bee Farms: YSOrganic.com
Z Natural Foods: ZNaturalFoods.com

Supplements

Dragon Herbs: DragonHerbs.com
From God's Pharmacy: FromGodsPharmacy.com
Gaia Herbs: GaiahHerbs.com
Garden of Life: GardenofLife.com
Green Foods: GreenFoods.com
Green Pasture: Greenpasture.org
Host Defense Mushrooms: HostDefense.com
iHerb: iHerb.com
Jing Herbs: JingHerbs.com
Jordan Rubin and Get Real Nutrition: iHerb.com
New Chapter: NewChapter.com
Nordic Naturals: NordicNaturals.com
Organic India: OrganicIndia.com
The Raw Food World: TheRawFoodWorld.com
Sisters of the Valley: Sistersofcbd.com
Terry Naturally Vitamins: Terrynaturally.com
Whole Body Research: WholeBodyResearch.com

Sweeteners, Coconut Nectar, Sugar, Stevia, Raw Honey, Maple Syrup

Big Tree Farms: BigTreeFarms.com
David Wolfe NoniLand Gold Honey: davidwolfe.com
Hidden Springs Maple Syrup: HiddenSpringsMaple.com
Longevity Warehouse: LongevityWarehouse.com
Madhava Sweeteners: MadhavaSweeteners.com
Maple Valley Cooperative: MapleValleySyrup.com
Now: NowFoods.com
Nuna Naturals: NunaNatural.com
Quarry Hill Farm Maple Syrup: QuarryHillFarmMaple.com
Really Raw Honey: ReallyRawHoney.com
Royal Kenyon Beeworks: KenyonBee.com

SweetLeaf: Sweetleaf.com (pure green leaf stevia)
Woodstock: Woodstock-Foods.com

Tea/Coffee
The Bean Organic Coffee Company: TheBeanCoffeeCompany.
  com
Dean's Beans: DeansBeans.com
The Fair Trade Coffee Company: FairTradeCoffee.org
Jim's Organic Coffee: JimsOrganicCoffee.com
Longevity Warehouse: LongevityWarehouse.com
Mighty Leaf: MightyLeaf.com
Newman's Own: NewmansOwn.com
Numi Organic Tea: numitea.com
The Organic Coffee Co.: OrganicCoffeeCompany.com
Organic India: OrganicIndia.com
The Republic of Tea: RepublicofTea.com (USDA organic only)
Seven Farms: SevenFarms.com
Subtle Earth Organic Coffee: cafedonpablo.com
Tazo: Tazo.com (USDA organic only)
Traditional Medicinals: TraditionalMedicinals.com
Yogi Tea: YogiTea.com

Tomato Sauces
Bionaturae: Bionaturae.com
Eden Foods: EdenFoods.com
Jovial: JovialFoods.com
Muir Glen Organic: MuirGlen.com
Woodstock: Woodstock-Foods.com

Veggie Burgers
Hillary's: HillarysEatWell.com
Sunshine Burgers: SunshineBurger.com

Vinegar/Seasonings
Bragg: Bragg.com
Coconut Secret: CoconutSecret.com

Wild Fish
Alaskan Seafood Market: TannersFish.com
The Little Fish Company: WildLittleFish.com
Tropical Traditions: TropicalTraditions.com
Wild Local Seafood: WildLocalSeafood.com

Yogurt and Kefir
Brown Cow: BrownCowFarm.com
Kalona Super Natural: KalonaSuperNatural.com
Kefir Lady: KefirLady.com
Maple Hill Creamery: MapleHillCreamery.com
Redwood Hill Farm and Creamery: RedwoodHill.com
Stonyfield Organic: Stonyfield.com

PERSONAL CARE PRODUCTS

Essential Oils
Aura Cacia: AuraCacia.com
dōTERRA: doterra.com
Dr. Axe (search for Numa Essential Oils Kit): Store.DrAxe.com
Mountain Rose Herbs: MountainRoseHerbs.com
Now: NowFoods.com
Plant Therapy: PlantTherapy.com
RMO (Rocky Mountain Oils): RockyMountainOils.com
Tropical Traditions: TropicalTraditions.com
Young Living: YoungLiving.com

Feminine Care
Natracare: Natracare.com

Hair Care Products
Aubrey Organics: AubreyOrganics.com
Avalon Organics: AvalonOrganics.com
Beyond Organic: MyBeyondOrganic.com
Dr. Organic: DrOrganic.com.uk
Hask: HaskBeauty.com
Juice Beauty: JuiceBeauty.com
Kiehls: Kiels.com
Miessence Certified Organics: Miessence.com
Natural Is Better: naturalisbetter.co.uk
Yarok LLC: Shop.Yarokhair.com
Young Living: YoungLiving.com

Hair Color
Hairprint: MyHairprint.com
Hennalucent: Store.GoldenMartBeautySupply.com
Heratint: Herbatint.co.uk
Naturtint: Naturtintusa.com
Light Mountain: Light-Mountain-Hair-Color.com
Tints of Nature: TintsofNature.com

Hand Soap, Bar Soap
Annanda Chaga: AnnandaChaga.com
Desert Essence: DesertEssence.com
Dr. Bronner's All-One!: DrBronner.com
The Grandpa Soap Co.: GrandpaSoap.com
The Honest Company: Honest.com
Kiss My Face: KissMyFace.com
Mrs. Meyer's: MrsMeyers.com

Nubian Heritage: NubianHeritage.com
One With Nature: OnewithNature.com (Dead Sea soap)
One Green Planet: OneGreenPlanet.com
Vermont Soap: VermontSoap.com

Makeup, Deodorant, Body Care, Sunscreen
Aubrey Organics: AubreyOrganics.com
Crystal: TheCrystal.com
Juice Beauty: JuiceBeauty.com
Dr. Hauschka: Dr.Hauschka.com
Dr. Mercola: Shop.Mercola.com
EB Ecco Bella: Eccobella.com
Miessence: Miessence.com
100% Pure: 100PercentPure.com
Poofy Organics: PoofyOrganics.com
Pure and True Organic Beauty: PureandTrue.com
Rejuva Minerals: RejuvaMinerals.com

Nail Polish, Nontoxic
Acquarella: Acquarella.com/collections/nail-polish
Honeybee Gardens: HoneybeeGardens.com
Peacekeeper: IAmaPeacekeeper.com
Piggy Paint: PiggyPaint.com
SpaRitual: SpaRitual.com

Skin Care, Dry Brushes, Loofah
BathEssential: BathEssential.com
Birchbox: Birchbox.com
The Body Shop: TheBodyShop.com.au
Desert Essence: DesertEssence.com
Dr. Bronner's All-One!: DrBronners.com
The Raw Food World: TheRawFoodWorld.com

The Organic Pharmacy: TheOrganicPharmacy.com
Tropical Traditions: TropicalTraditions.com
Weleda: Weleda.com
Yerba Primer: Yerba.com

Teeth Care, Fluoride-Free
Desert Essence: Desertessence.com
Earthpaste: Earthpaste.com
Miessence: Miessence.com
Nature's Gate: NaturesGate.com
Weleda: Weleda.com
Dr. Bronner's All-One!: Drbronner.com

DETERGENTS AND PAPER PRODUCTS

Detergents, Laundry and Dish
CitraSolv: CitraSolv.com
Ecover: Ecover.com
Greenshield Organic: GreenshieldOrganic.com
The Honest Company: Honest.com
Mrs. Meyer's: MrsMeyers.com
Planet: PlanetInc.com
Seventh Generation: SeventhGeneration.com
Tropical Traditions: TropicalTraditions.com

Paper Products
Chasing Green: ChasingGreen.org
If You Care: IfYouCare.com
Natural Value: NaturalValue.com
Seventh Generation: SeventhGeneration.com

APPLIANCES

Blenders, Juicers, and Food Processors
Breville: Breville.com
Hurom: Hurom.com
Jack LaLanne's Power Juicer: PowerJuicer.com
Juicepresso: Juicepressousa.com
KitchenAid: KitchenAid.com
Norwalk: NorwalkJuicers.com
Nutribullet: Nutribullet.com
Rawfully Organic Coop: RawfullyOrganic.com
Tropical Traditions: TropicalTraditions.com
Vitamix: Vitamix.com

Frying Pans, Pots, and Baking Pans
Chalphalon: Chalphalon.com
Cuisineart: CuisinartWebstore.com
Dr. Mercola: Cookware.mercola.com
Emile Henry: EmileHenryusa.com
Fox Run Brands: FoxRunBrands.com
GreenPan: Greenpan.us
Heim Concept: HeimConcept.com
Lodge Cast Iron: Lodgemfg.com
Miriam's Earthen Cookware: MiriamsEarthenCookware.com

Pressure and Slow Cookers
Presto: Gopresto.com
Cuisine Pressure Cooker Recipes: CuisinartPressureCooker-
    recipes.blogspot.com
Prestige Smart Kitchen: PrestigeSmartKitchen.com
VitaClayChef: VitaClayChef.com

Coffee Makers, Nontoxic

Breville: Brevilleusa.com
Chemex: ChemexCoffeemaker.com
The Coffee Concierge: TheCoffeeConcierge.net
Hamilton Beach: HamiltonBeach.com
Primula: PrimulaProducts.com
WestBend: Westbend.com

Coffee Filters, Nontoxic

Chemex: ChemexCoffeemaker.com
Houzz: Houzz.com
If You Care: IfYouCare.com

Green Flatware, Cups, and Plates

Earth 911: Earth911.com

Organic Produce/Organic, Heirloom Seeds

Cascadian Farm Organic: CascadianFarm.com
Driscoll's: Driscolls.com
Earthbound Farm: EarthboundFarm.com
Eden Brothers: EdenBrothers.com (organic seeds)
Farmbox Direct: FarmboxDirect.com
Olivia's Organics: OliviasOrganics.org
Organic Seed Alliance: SeedAlliance.org
Seed Savers Exchange: SeedSavers.org
Sproutman: Sproutman.com
Sprout People: SproutPeople.org
Taylor Farms: TaylorFarms.com
Woodstock: Woodstock-Foods.com

Pet Food

Amore Pet Foods: AmorePetFoods.com

Cat Connection: CatConnection.com (Wild Side Salmon
freeze-dried treats)

Dog Food Advisor: Dogfoodadvisor.com

Darwin's Natural Pet Products: DarwinsPet.com

Newman's Own: NewmansOwn.com

Rebounders

Vuly: VulyTrampolines.us

Water Sources, Filters, and Drinking Water

Aclare Waterwise: HealthyPerceptions.com

Beyond Organic: BeyondOrganic.com

Dr. Mercola: Waterfilters.Mercola.com/products.asp

Enviro Products: NewWaveEnviro.com

Evamor: Evamor.com

Fiji Water: FijiWater.com

Locate a Spring: FindaSpring.com

Bibliography

American Chemical Society (ACS) (2016). "Curious crystals."
Available at http://www.inquiryinaction.org/
chemistryreview/solids/

Axe, J. (January 2015). "Is agave nectar good for you?" Dr.
Axe: Food Is Medicine. Available at https://draxe.
com/agave-nectar/

Blaylock, Russell L. 1994. *Excitotoxins: the taste that kills.* Santa
Fe, N.M.: Health Press.

Brown, T. (January 2014). "Natural vs. synthetic vitamins."
Georgia Health Solutions. Available at http://
georgiahealthsolutions.com/2014/01/

Enig, M., & Fallon, S. (August 2002). "The truth about
saturated fat." Mercola. Available at http://articles.
mercola.com/sites/articles/archive/2002/08/17/
saturated-fat1.aspx

Gardener, H., et al. (2012). "Diet soft drink consumption is
associated with an increased risk of vascular events."
NCBI. Available at https://www.ncbi.nlm.nih.gov/
pubmed/22282311

Group, E. (2016). "The differences between synthetic and
natural vitamins." Global Healing Center. Available at
http://www.globalhealingcenter.com/natural-health/
synthetic-vs-natural-vitamins/

Health Benefits of Noni Juice (n.d.). Organic Facts. Available
at https://www.organicfacts.net/health-benefits/
beverage/noni-juice.html

Herring, K. (February 26, 2014). "The hidden danger in your slow cooker." Wellness Blog. Available at http://blog.grasslandbeef.com/bid/89368/The-Hidden-Danger-in-Your-Slow-Cooker

Huff, E. (July 2014). "Sucralose vs. aspartame: Which of these top two artificial sweeteners is the better choice?" Natural News. Available at http://www.naturalnews.com/045824_sucralose_aspartame_artificial_sweeteners.html

International Olive Oil Council (n.d.). "The differences between virgin olive oil (VOO) and extra-virgin olive oil (EVOO) and fine virgin olive oil." CureZone. Available at http://www.curezone.org/cleanse/liver/oliveoil.asp

Jenkins, O. (February 2014). "A step-by-step guide to dry brushing." MBG: MindBodyGreen. Available at http://www.mindbodygreen.com/0-12675/a-step-by-step-guide-to-dry-skin-brushing.html

Jockers, D. (April 2011). "Be informed: Nonstick pans pose danger." Natural News. Available at http://www.naturalnews.com/031946_nonstick_cookware_health_danger.html

Jong, N. (December 2014). "10 healthy reasons to drink coffee." One Medical. Available at http://www.onemedical.com/blog/newsworthy/10-healthy-reasons-to-drink-coffee-2/

Marson, A. (April 2014). "Colossal coconut oil." Mature Living Toledo. Available at http://digital.zoompubs.com/article/Colossal+Coconut+Oil/1675492/0/article.html

Martinez, K. "What is olive oil? What are the differences?" Antonio Celentano Extra Virgin Olive Oil. Available at http://www.real-restaurant-recipes.com/olive-oil-article.html

Mayo Clinic Staff (December 2016). "Lead poisoning." Available at http://www.mayoclinic.org/diseases-conditions/lead-poisoning/home/ovc-20275050

MDidea (2014). "The History of the Olive Tree" MDidea Pure Herbal Extracts. Available at https://www.mdidea. com/products/proper/proper06208.html

Mercola, J. (August 2010). "The cholesterol myth that is harming your health." Mercola. Available at http://articles.mercola. com/sites/articles/archive/2010/08/10/ making-sense-of-your-cholesterol-numbers.aspx?i_ cid=cse-tbd-cholesterol-content

Naidenko, O., Leiga, N., Skharp, R., & Houlihan, J. (2008). "Bottled water contains disinfection byproducts, fertilizer residue, and pain medication." EWG: The Environmental Working Group. Available at http:// www.ewg.org/research/bottled-water-quality-investigation

Omics International (2014). "Ghee." Available at http:// research.omicsgroup.org/index.php/Ghee

Paige, E. (September 2013). "Raw milk benefits and song." Health Banquet. Available at http://www. healthbanquet.com/raw-milk.html

Price, W. (2010). *Nutrition and physical degeneration: A comparison of primitive and modern diets and their effects.* Oxford, UK: Benediction Classics.

Ranasinghe, P., Pigera, S., Sirimal Premakurmara, G. A., Galappaththy, P., Constantine, G. R., & Katulanda, P. (2013). "Medicinal properties of 'true' cinnamon: A systematic review." BMC Complementary and Alternative Medicine. Available at https://bmccomplementalternmed.biomedcentral.com/articles/10.1186/1472-6882-13-275

Rogers, S. (1994). *Wellness against all odds.* Solvay, NY: Prestige.

Rosso, S. Sera F, Segnan N. Zanetti R. (2008). "Sun exposure prior to diagnosis is associated with improved survival in melanoma patients: Results from a long-term follow-up study of Italian patients." NCBI. Available at https://www.ncbi.nlm.nih.gov/pubmed/18406602

Rubin, J. S. (2004). *The maker's diet: The 40-day health experience that will change your life forever.* Shippensburg, PA: Destiny Image.

Szekely, E. (Ed. and Trans.) (1981). *The Essene gospel of peace, Book I.* Nelson, BC, Canada: International Biogenic Society.

Wolfe, D. (February 2013). "Superfoods list and top tips from David Wolfe." Superfood Blog. Available at http://superfoodblog.co.uk/superfoods-list-and-top-tips-from-david-wolfe/

About the Author

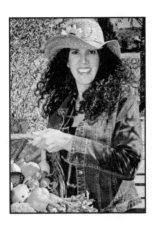

Tonijean Kulpinski lives with her husband of twenty-five years; her beautiful daughter, Michaela; and her lovely golden retriever, Peanut. Toni is a Board-Certified Holistic Practitioner, a Certified Biblical Health Coach, a member of The American Association of Drugless Practitioners, and The Weston Price Foundation. Tonijean is a graduate of The Institute for Integrative Nutrition, the world's largest nutrition school. She is the owner of Heaven on Earth Healing Center, Inc., where she dedicates her private practice to educating patients how to stop battling disease and start building wellness.

Toni also teaches holistic nutrition for adult enrichment at The Desmond Campus of Mount Saint Mary's College, a well-known university located in Newburgh, New York. For the past six years, she has appeared on TBN's *Joy in Our Town* and *Doctor to Doctor*, televised from The Manhattan Studio.

Tonijean bases her teaching on principles stated clearly in scripture and has learned from her own health experience that food in the form God created is the medicine that heals. She is on her God-given mission to help transform the health of this nation and world with the truth revealed in nature's medicine and the connection inside every human.

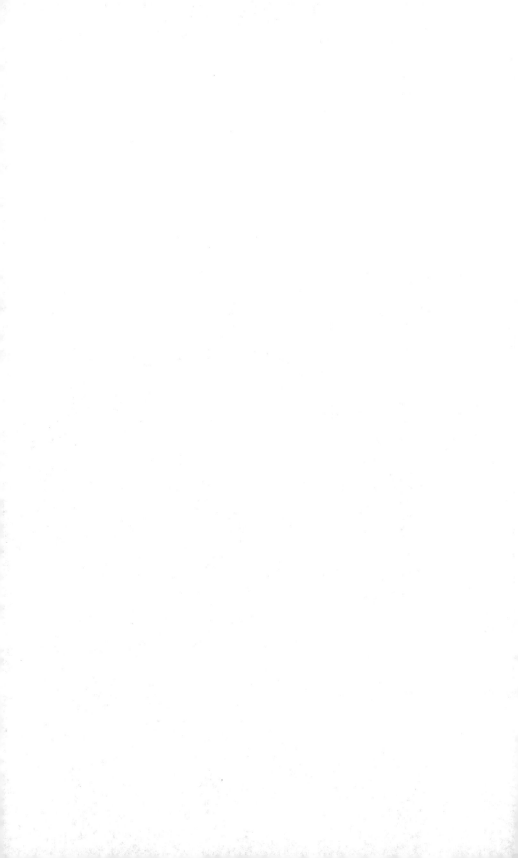